Baby steps and gold stars

'*How to Eat Loads and Stay Slim*' really is different - it's not a diet book. This bears repeating: *This is not a diet book.* It doesn't promise the world, but it *does* promise change - a bit at a time (and let's face it, a 'bit' is all the change you or I are willing to make).

How does it happen? With a simple 'gold star' system. Read the chapter, make one or two (teeny) changes at the end, and gain a star.

It's simple and effective. No magic, no false promises, just sound advice from people who have been where you are. And, little by little, things start changing.

Nicola McKenna, 19 August 2013

Common sense means no more dieting

Great book that takes a common sense approach to dieting. You'll learn about sensible snacks, healthy eating and why the body craves things the way it does. I was particularly intrigued by the "oil diet", which I might have to try some time. I love the way the book alternates between Peter's *fry-up* attitude and Dellas more healthy salad and soup approach- something for everyone. Definitely worth reading- this is a book I will keep referring back to.

'BlueCat', 24 May 2013

A Good Guide!

No-nonsense and sensible eating practices, with a few tips and tricks thrown in that I hadn't heard of before.

Mr P J Grant, 10 Jun 2013

Sound Common Sense and Entertaining read too

This book was very entertaining. I laughed out loud at some of the sections. The authors are very funny. It was also full of helpful advice. Basically, make a lot of small changes to make a big change to your weight. No hardship to read it, and not really a hardship to make the changes.

I thought the idea of a fatometer was hilarious.

If you've got a good sense of humour you will love this book. I thoroughly recommend it to anyone who is struggling with their weight and doesn't want to starve for two days a week. Excellent stuff.

Amazon Customer, 11 Jun 2013

Makes sense, and made me laugh too

Having yo-yo dieted my whole life, I've finally found a book (not a diet!) that has inspired me to get the weight off and be able to keep it off. The authors remind me throughout that life doesn't revolve around a diet, but that healthy eating is an easy lifestyle choice. The book is packed with humour and the authors differing yet similar views in relation to eating made me belly laugh at times, and I am anticipating a smaller belly soon! Buy this book if you are fed up with dieting, I will never use the words "I'm on a diet" again!

A M Rutland, 28 May 2013

Read more 5-star reviews at amazon.co.uk,
and also at
HowToEatLoadsAndStaySlim.com

How To Eat Loads and Stay Slim

**Your diet-free guide
to losing weight
without feeling hungry!**

Peter Jones & Della Galton

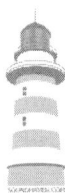

soundhaven books
www.soundhaven.com

Published 2014 in Great Britain,
by soundhaven books
http://www.soundhaven.com

Please visit
www.howtoeatloadsandstayslim.com
for contact details

ISBN: 978-0-9568856-1-6

British Cataloguing Publication data:
A catalogue record of this book is available from
the British Library

This book is also available as an ebook, and in audio.
Please visit
www.howtoeatloadsandstayslim.com
for more details.

To Wendy,
For all your love & support.
May you never need to worry about anything,
least of all your weight,
Peter

For Adam, who doesn't need to worry about his weight,
but is gorgeous enough as he is.
With love,
Della

Contents

Foreword

By Dr Karen King FRSA,
also known as novelist Catherine King

Catherine Says...

Most of my readers know that I was a lecturer before I became a full-time author, but not many are aware that prior to my lecturing career I was a State Registered Dietician at The Addenbrookes Hospital in Cambridge. Therefore I have a knowledgeable interest in scientific developments surrounding nutrition and health, especially those concerning appetite control. In addition, I have recently lost over 30 pounds of excess weight. These two things alone qualify me to write this foreword and recommend that you read Della and Peter's wise guide based on their personal experiences. However, there is another reason why this book makes so much sense to me.

During the latter part of my academic career I operated as a change agent, contributing to the management of change in several UK universities. This book is about change – change for the better. My personal weight loss is primarily due to change. I have changed the way I shop, I have changed the way I cook and, therefore, I have changed the way I eat. Della and Peter explain how you can change based on their own similar successes. It is a survival guide for keeping your weight under control in our present-day unhelpful eating environment. Read it and try it for yourself.

Best wishes
Catherine King

Find out more about Catherine and all her other books at www.catherineking.info

To Begin With…

Peter Says…

When I was a much younger man, the only pounds I ever had to worry about were the ones that should have been in my wallet. 'Fat' wasn't a word that was ever used in connection with me. I was the living embodiment of 'tall' and 'skinny'.

Even in my twenties, when I was mostly living on a diet of pizza and beer, where most people have a 'bottom' I had a 'place where my legs met'. Girls would tell me how lucky I was. Guys would question my ability to lift a bag of sugar. I'd just shrug, convinced that I'd never lose my ability to hide behind lamp posts or squeeze between railings.

How wrong I was.

I met my wife-to-be in my mid-thirties. The fact that I met Kate at all was something of a minor miracle, but her arrival in my life coincided with another miraculous event: I'd started to put on weight.

In a matter of months I somehow went from ten stone eight (148 pounds) to thirteen stone (182 pounds). People started to tell me how 'well' I looked. Occasionally I was described as 'cuddly'. And as Kate and I curled up in front of the TV to munch our way through a family sized bar of chocolate, she'd rub what she fondly referred to as the 'Buddha Belly'. It was almost enough to ruin my appetite.

Almost – but not quite.

As the months passed my weight crept ever upwards. My chins (plural) got ever bigger. Eventually I no longer felt comfortable being naked in front of my fiancé.

And that was the turning point.

Not the naked part – the fact that my girlfriend was now my fiancée. And on hearing the happy news one of my colleagues asked me when I was starting my diet.

"Diet?!" I asked, with a mixture of indignation and confusion. What had diets got to do with marriage?

"Of course diet," she said. "You're never as slim as the day you get married!"

This was news to me, and something of a shock. And although the logical, adult part of my brain was quick to dismiss this as utter nonsense, another part – the part that has always been ready to believe anything negative or damaging – had already adopted this as a Universal Truth. I had only a few months to lose those pounds that I still thought of as 'extra' – or they would be mine *forever*. The clock was ticking.

It was nonsense, of course. But you've been there, I'm sure. Bouncing from one diet to another in an effort to avoid what seems to be the inevitable – 'you will never be as slim as you once were'. Maybe you're at that point now, in which case you're probably familiar with a couple of other 'Universal Truths', namely that diets and exercise are miserable, soul destroying ways of losing weight, and if you stop either one for a millisecond then those grams that you worked so hard to shed come straight back the moment you so much as look at anything vaguely tasty.

There are few things in this life as cruel as how the human body manages its weight. At least that's how it feels. And I don't know about you, but there's only so much heartache I can take. After a couple of years of running in my lunch hour – returning to my desk hot, frustrated, and not the slightest bit lighter than the day before (or the week before, or any of the preceding months) – I finally threw my heart-rate monitor in the bin and went in search of a pain-free, exercise-free, scientific way to restore my trim figure.

This book – or at least my half of it – is the result.

Welcome to How To Eat Loads and Stay Slim.

If you're fed up with diets – this book might be for you.

If you've started to wonder whether you'll ever be able to lose weight, stay slim AND enjoy your food – this book is probably for you.

But if you're open minded, happy to make several small changes to your lifestyle, and prepared to put in a little effort – or at least could be, if you had a good enough reason – then this book is most definitely for you.

Now then, allow me to introduce you to my co-author…

Della Says…

Like Peter, I am lucky enough to be tall, almost six foot, and until I was thirty-five, which, incidentally, is also the age I was when I got married – must be something in this 'marry-and-get-fat' theory – I was pretty slender without putting too much effort into it. Mind you, I had always been very active. I loved to go swimming and running and having four dogs certainly helped to keep my weight down.

Then suddenly I had a husband who was a foodie, which meant we ate out a lot and had wine with most of our meals and I began to experiment with cooking rich food. Not that I objected to any of this! But slowly the weight inched on. I went from being a skinny size twelve to a cuddlier size sixteen. This doesn't sound too bad; it didn't look too bad either because I'm tall, but I hated my extra weight with a vengeance.

I began to dress to cover up lumps and bumps. Big loose tops and black trousers became my uniform. I gave up swimming because I didn't want my cellulite thighs on display on the walk from changing room to pool. I avoided hugging friends I hadn't seen for a while so they couldn't feel how much weight I'd put on, which is terribly sad now I stop to think about it. I gave up clothes shopping because it was too depressing. Nothing looked good any more.

Choosing an outfit for a night out was hideously depressing and would entail trying on my entire wardrobe – by this time I had three sizes in there, size twelve (dream on!), size fourteen (possibly on a good day) and size sixteen (comfortably unflattering) – and trying to decide what made me look the thinnest.

I'd always felt self-conscious about being tall, but being tall and overweight made it worse. I felt as though I was turning into some huge lumbering hippo.

My mother and sister also struggled with their weight. My mother had given up worrying about it long ago; my sister, like me, had yo-yoed along, losing weight only to pile it back on again.

In my quest for permanent weight loss I tried the following:

➢   slimming pills
➢   herbal remedies
➢   crash diets
➢   small portions
➢   not eating in the evenings
➢   not eating certain foods
➢   various celebrity diets
➢   some decidedly cranky diets
➢   slimming groups
➢   excessive exercise – and I mean running marathons (I don't do things by halves).

Nothing worked long term.

I lost half a stone, I gained half a stone, and usually a few more pounds besides, and the older I got the harder this battle became. My half a stone turned into a stone and then two, which was doubly difficult to shift. Clearly something had to be done, but I didn't know what.

Then one day, after I'd lost the same two stone for the umpteenth time and was waiting for the pounds to inevitably pile back on again I had a eureka moment.

The answer to being slim, I finally realised, was to stick to a variety of tried and tested principles. *My* tried and tested principles which had worked for me. To my immense relief and pleasure, these principles did not include banishing any food from my life. They required planning, but they weren't time consuming (I have no spare time in my life), and they weren't costly (I spend all my spare money on dogs).

But they do work. Hurrah! Finally, I am the same weight now as I was when I was twenty and I know how to stay there. And it is much, much more enjoyable. I also feel healthier, which is a big bonus. And I don't worry if I go on holiday and put on a few pounds because I know it won't be difficult to shift them again.

If this sounds like it might suit you then read on – and hopefully some of the concepts we talk about in this book might change the way you view staying slim too.

How To Eat Loads and Stay Slim

(Peter says...)

There are certain things in this world which just aren't up for debate.

For instance, contrary to what people may have thought the world is spherical in shape. It's certainly not flat. Every three hundred and sixty five days – or thereabouts – it makes a journey around the sun. Very few people still think our planet is the centre of the universe. And whilst there are parts of the world where this isn't the case, for the vast majority of us the sun rises each morning, and sets each night. These things are called 'facts'. 'Truths' that make up the fabric of the universe.

Here are some other 'facts' you might be familiar with: Anything that tastes nice is probably fattening. Being slim is mostly genetic, or a 'young person' thing. Some people can eat anything without putting on weight. You're not one of those people. And my personal favourite...

YOU CAN EAT LOADS,
OR STAY SLIM.
YOUR CHOICE.

But then, if any of those were remotely true either my size or my meals choices would be making me unhappy

– and I'm completely happy with both. What's more, my bathroom scales wouldn't be buried at the back of a cupboard somewhere. And you wouldn't be holding this book.

The reality is, you really can eat loads and stay slim.

Let's start by giving you some new 'truths'.

Basic Principles

(Della says…)

There are Seven Basic Principles that underpin How To Eat Loads and Stay Slim.

PRINCIPLE NUMBER 1:
EAT LOADS

I love food. So does Peter. For us and many other people out there – including you, I suspect – eating is a joy. And when we came up with the title for this book, 'eat loads' was supposed to reflect our enthusiasm of enjoying really tasty food. It wasn't (as many people have suggested) some sort of reference to the quantities of lettuce you must consume if you want to stay slim. That would be no fun at all! Not unless it was smothered in a very tasty dressing. Maybe a few sesame seeds thrown in for good measure, a small dollop of full fat mayo on the side… are you feeling hungry yet?

Before we started writing this book, before we'd even met, Peter and I had independently come to the conclusion that any weight loss solution that compromised our enjoyment of food was never going to work. Not for us. And probably not for you.

Whilst we're not about to suggest you stuff your face with burgers every meal time, or skip meals entirely and live on chocolate bars, we firmly believe that whatever you put in your mouth has to be nice, and you have to be able to eat lots of it.

PRINCIPLE NUMBER 2:
STAY SLIM

Let me tell you something you already know: losing weight is hard work. And it can be soul destroying – particularly as it's often about not doing things – not eating what you want, for example, whilst you wait – patiently, impatiently – for that flab to disappear, which for some ungodly reason takes far longer than it took to appear in the first place.

Losing weight really is about 'losing', and nobody likes to lose.

Which is why this isn't a weight loss book.

Sure, if you have a few extra pounds, maybe more than a few, we can help you to shed those and then some, but mostly this book is about making smarter choices – choices that'll make it almost impossible to be anything other than slim.

PRINCIPLE NUMBER 3:
DIETS DON'T WORK

The problem with diets – all diets, even the weird one mentioned later in this book – is that they're temporary. Stick to the diet and you'll lose weight; come off the diet and the weight you lost will find its way home again. If the problem that diets are trying to solve is "how do I lose weight and keep it off?" then dieting isn't actually the solution.

So what is?

The answer, of course, is permanent, long term changes. *Change your diet*, rather than *go on a diet.* Which leads me rather nicely onto Basic Principle Number 4.

PRINCIPLE NUMBER 4:
YOU HAVE TO CHANGE

There are those of you who will read this book, finish it …and do absolutely nothing else.

And that won't work.

Sorry about that.

The fact is, if you want to eat loads and stay slim, you're going to have to change *something*.

PRINCIPLE NUMBER 5:
MAKE MANY, MANY
IMPERCEPTIBLE CHANGES

The good news is that the 'changes' you need to make don't have to be huge. A tweak here and another tweak there will steadily make it less and less possible for you to be anything other than slim, whilst allowing you to maintain a love of meal times.

PRINCIPLE NUMBER 6:
HEALTHY EATING,
MOST OF THE TIME,
IS USUALLY GOOD ENOUGH

Now don't do that.

Don't try and deny it. I saw you.

You rolled your eyes!

Peter and I are not going to suggest that you stop eating burgers, or pizza, or chips, or anything else. We are, however, going to help you make those foods healthier. Or space out those convenient, comforting meals with other great tasting foods. We want to get you to a point where, on the whole, the stuff you put in your mouth is both tasty and good for you.

All of which will take some effort.

Which is why you need the final Basic Principle.

PRINCIPLE NUMBER 7:
PLAN.
(IF YOU FAIL TO PLAN
YOU'VE PLANNED TO FAIL)

The final and most basic of principles in our quest to help you eat loads and stay slim is *planning*. We're not going to ask you to fill out charts, but some thinking on your part, much of it of the 'forward thinking' variety, will be required. If you can organise yourself to moderate degree – if you can make a list or two, know your way around a calendar, or set a reminder on your phone – effective weight management is well within your grasp.

But before you start purchasing wall charts or anything similar, I'd like you to think about 'stars'.

Stars & Action Points

(Peter says…)

The problem with many self-help books, in my experience, is that the advice they contain is usually a lot easier to read than heed. You'll sit there, chuckling away, occasionally saying to yourself "That's a good idea" – then you'll turn the page.

Before you know it you're at the end of the book, and no slimmer than when you started.

Don't do that.

Throughout this book you'll come across various 'Action Points'. These boxes serve as Stop Signs – the idea is that you stop, address the action, and then continue.

Now clearly if you ignore the Action Point – the Stop Sign – it's unlikely that you'll be hit by a truck a moment later. I'm not going to pursue you through the following pages, flag you down and issue you with a ticket and 3 points on your library card. But I have some bad news for you: reading this book without any kind of follow up action won't have the effect you're looking for.

Remember Basic Principle Number Four:

PRINCIPLE NUMBER 4:
YOU HAVE TO CHANGE

Nobody likes change. As human beings we're pretty much hardwired to try and 'stay the same', and resist anything that represents change. Sometimes it's astonishing how hard we'll resist change, regardless of how good the alternative is.

But by the same token, sometimes it's the strangest little things that can motivate us.

I'm not just an author. To two people in this world, my primary job is that of 'Uncle'. I take this role very seriously. It's kind of a cross between being a clown, a punch bag, an audience, and a confidante.

I remember one weekend when my nephew and niece were six. Whilst my niece was her usual non-stop-chatty self, my nephew spent much of the time with his face in a book. And not just a book, but a bumper book of maths puzzles. He spent the weekend doing sums.

Was he catching up on school homework?

No – he bought the book with his own pocket money.

Did his parents encourage him to work through the book by way of some extra study?

No – it was completely voluntary.

Why then had he chosen to spend his time in this way?

Because of the stars.

At the back of my nephew's book there were several sheets of self-adhesive gold stars, and at the bottom of each page was space for a gold star to be stuck once the page had been completed. This simple concept very much appealed to my young nephew.

Della and I think that it might just work for you.

Now unfortunately there are no stars at the back of this book, nor a place for you to stick them if there were. Our stars are imaginary. Sorry about that. They are, however, much more powerful.

There are fifty four stars available. You've already earned one just for buying this book (see the front cover), and with every additional star you acquire you will steadily increase your chances of being able to eat loads AND stay slim. Collect enough stars (thirty or more would be a good target to have) and we personally guarantee that a slim figure, coupled with a healthy but satiated appetite, are yours for the taking. And all you have to do to earn a star is complete an action point.

You bought this book because something in your head said "Hey – I *do* want to eat loads and stay slim". With all that in mind then here's your second star and first Action Point of the book.

STOP! ACTION POINT!

Commit to making changes

WORTH ONE STAR

Make a promise to yourself right now that *this time* you'll follow some advice, and you'll do the actions – most of them, anyway – as we go along.

Make the promise out loud, tell a friend, say it in your head, I don't care – just do it.

Now.

Done it?

Ok. Well done.

You have another star.

How Hunger *Really* Works

(Peter says…)

Two stars already, eh? That wasn't too difficult, was it, and already you're another step closer to being a more slender you. One step closer to being an 'Eat-Loadser'. Get you! How d'you feel? Excited? Nervous? Sceptical? Empowered? Hungry?

Whoops – sorry, I didn't mean hungry. That just slipped in there. But isn't that always the way? There you are, in a high powered business meeting, nodding sagely whilst your client tells you how they're just not getting the performance they expected out of the new system you sold them, and all you can think about is whether the canteen will still have any bacon rolls when you're done.

There's a whole slew of weight management advice out there that can be summarised by the following sentence:

EAT WHEN YOU'RE HUNGRY

Fat people – so the proponents of this advice are keen to point out – will eat for numerous reasons other than hunger. They will eat when they're bored. They will eat when they're sad. Or because it's lunchtime. Or out of habit. Or because they're thirsty. Or because there's still food on the plate. Or in the fridge. Or in the shop.

The 'eat when you're hungry' advice generally makes a lot of sense – unless you genuinely feel hungry a lot of the time, then it's a recipe (pardon the pun) for disaster.

Enter another slew of weight loss gurus for whom the following is their mantra:

IT'S OK TO FEEL HUNGRY.
FEELING HUNGRY IS NORMAL.

These people want you to make friends with your hunger pangs. Accept them as part of the norm. Know that being hungry doesn't necessarily mean starvation is just around the corner. Which is all well and good, of course, if you're one of those people who can mentally push hunger to one side. Personally if I'm hungry I can't concentrate on anything properly until I've shoved something tasty in 'me gob'. And if – God forbid – there's no food available I'm likely to gnaw off my arm.

And isn't that how it's supposed to be? Surely hunger – like pain – is a natural reaction designed to motivate us into taking action? If it isn't then why on earth do we get hungry?

That is a very, very good question.

Why Your Body Makes You Hungry

(Peter says…)

Many, many years ago, long before you and I came to be – before the invention of the internet, the telephone, pizza delivery services, before mopeds, and the wheels that make them possible – before anyone had even thought of taking a slab of pizza dough, smothering it in tomato paste and putting cheese on top – food was generally hard to come by. The only meal options available were fruit, nuts and berries – or catching something and killing it. Which could be a tad treacherous and usually involved a joint effort. Times were tough.

This being the case, it didn't really make a lot of sense to evolve a hunger mechanism that made your tummy rumble just because you hadn't eaten. Not when there just wasn't any food available, and the first pizza delivery company wouldn't be around for several thousand years.

On the other hand, when food was plentiful – say, when your old pal Ug had managed to trap a woolly mammoth – it made a LOT of sense for your body to encourage you to eat as much as you could from the all-you-can-eat mammoth buffet, because tomorrow that woolly mammoth might be past its 'best slaughtered by' date and you'd be back foraging amongst the bushes. In those days, life was quite often a case of 'survival of the fattest.'

Of course, back in the 21st century every day is 'woolly mammoth day'. Figuratively speaking. Food is plentiful, and quite a lot of it is packed with calories. And whilst we might eventually evolve a new hunger mechanism that takes all this into account, right now your body and mine are operating on the assumption that the local pizza delivery place might run out of pizza at any moment, and that it's best to fill up whilst we can.

Put simply, your body is designed to make you fatter.

Let's have a closer look at how it does that.

You Are Not A Car

(Peter says…)

If you're like me then you've probably gone through most of your life assuming that hunger is like the fuel warning light that some posh cars have – you're low on fuel, so you get hungry. Right?

No.

Being 'low on fuel' does indeed make you hungry, but how hungry you feel, and how often, is far from simple. You, dear reader, are quite a lot more sophisticated than even the poshest of posh road vehicles, and the mechanism that human beings have evolved to control hunger is really quite ingenious.

In 2005, Dr Seth Roberts (PhD) published a paper entitled "What Makes Food Fattening? A Pavlovian Theory of Weight Control"[1]. In it Dr Roberts cites a number of hitherto unconnected studies (mainly on rats) that led him to make several surprising conclusions, most of which run completely counter to what you and I 'know' – or think we know – about how our body works. Let's break them down:

---

[1] You'll find a link to Dr Roberts' paper on our website: howtoeatloadsandstayslim.com

Surprising conclusion number 1: "the body-fat set point"

To begin with Dr Roberts claims that the human body, yours and mine, has a built in "body-fat set-point" – a weight your body wants to be. I like to think of it as a 'fatometer'.

Your fatometer is a little like the central heating system in your house. Just as the heating goes on and off depending on how you've set your thermostat, your body will turn on hunger, or turn it off, make you feel full, or not, depending on whether you're lighter or heavier than the weight your fatometer is trying to achieve.

This sounds far-fetched, but in the last decade or so scientists have indeed discovered several hormones (Peptide Tyrosine Tyrosine (PYY), Ghrelin, Leptin… there are others) that control our hunger, appetite, and how quickly we feel satiated after eating. You've probably assumed you felt stuffed because there literally wasn't any room left in your stomach, and those hunger pangs were like the sound an empty oil drum makes when you beat it with a stick. Turns out those feelings are just feelings – they're 'chemical'.

Surprising conclusion number 2: what you eat changes your fatometer

The second intriguing element of Dr Roberts' paper is that just as your central heating's thermostat dial isn't fixed, neither is your body's fatometer. The body turns your fatometer up and down in direct response to what you eat, or don't eat. The more calories the body registers, the higher it sets your fatometer, and the more hungry you'll feel later.

So eat something really calorific – say, a slice of cake – and your body turns your fatometer way up, which kicks your overall appetite through the roof.

"How can that be?" you might be asking yourself. How can the body possibly know how many calories are in a slice of cake?

Surprising conclusion number 3: the body 'learns' how many calories your food has

Though we're totally unaware of it, each time we sit down to a meal our minds are busy consulting with our stomachs and associating the flavour of that meal with the calories it contains. Over time your body actually figures out which flavours have the most calories so that it can adjust your fatometer accordingly.

Of course this doesn't happen overnight, but as you might expect, foods that taste identical each and every time – such as a burger from a burger chain, or a pizza from a pizza delivery company, or your favourite chocolate bar – create very strong associations very quickly indeed.

Surprising conclusion number 4: Some foods turn down the fatometer

Finally, some good news. According to Doctor Roberts, if a food has calories, but your body hasn't created an association with its flavour, your body will actually turn down your fatometer, thereby lowering your appetite and causing you to feel more full when you eat.

So, for example, were you to sit down to a lovely plate of calorie-laden Ruurgh, which I'm reasonably certain you've never had before in your life (mainly because it's a dish I just made up), your body would turn _down_ your fatometer in response, which will lower your appetite for subsequent meals.

Now all this sciencey fatometer stuff can be, if you'll forgive the pun, a little hard to stomach. It's enough to make your head spin. So let me try and summarise it in one sentence.

THE MORE CALORIES YOU EAT,
AND THE MORE FAMILIAR YOUR FOOD,
THE HUNGRIER YOU'LL BECOME
AND THE MORE YOU'LL HAVE TO EAT TO FEEL FULL.

Turns out you are not a car.

You are much, much more complex.

Of course, this is all very interesting but what you really want to know is whether we can use this information to eat loads and stay slim? Is that possible?

Absolutely.

Knowing Your Enemy

(Peter says...)

Now that we know how the body works the world of weight gain – and, more importantly, weight loss – looks somewhat different. Let's take a closer look.

Why 'bad foods' are even worse for you than you originally thought

That bag of chips or a bar of chocolate doesn't make you put on weight just because they contain a lot of calories. The real problem is that your body has learnt to associate those calories with their yummy flavour, and will crank up your fatometer each time you eat them. This in turn makes you more and more hungry, which drives you to eat more. It's a weight gain double whammy!

High calorie-flavour foods are like those people who, when invited to a small, select cocktail party, rock up with a dozen or more rowdy mates. Pretty soon that party is out of control.

Why traditional diets are so difficult to follow

If you're overweight the chances are your fatometer is set really, really high, and 'cutting down' will be almost impossible. You'll be fighting a ravenous appetite that's part of a mechanism to make you eat when food's available.

The only way to extinguish that appetite is to eat foods that lower your fatometer.

Why home-cooked meals and a varied menu is better for you than anyone previously realised

'New' foods with new flavours, things you don't eat very often, home-cooked meals, vegetables – these foods won't turn your fatometer up as high as your favourite burger. If the food is completely unfamiliar to you your body might even turn your fatometer down, causing your overall appetite to fall.

In his book The Shangri-La Diet, Doctor Roberts mentions an intriguing study where a group of volunteers were asked to change the flavour of their food by seasoning their meals with a variety of ever changing random herbs and spices. This group ended up losing more weight over a six month period than a similar group on a standard calorie controlled diet.

Now don't tell me that that doesn't intrigue you. Even a little bit.

Let's integrate what we've learnt into our eating habits.

STOP! ACTION POINT!

Understanding your fatometer (body-weight set-point)

WORTH ONE STAR

Familiarise yourself with the science behind how hunger really works to claim one star:
- ➢ Your body has a fatometer which determines how fat your body wants to be.
- ➢ The fatometer controls hunger and how full you feel.
- ➢ The body learns how calorific your food is.
- ➢ Familiar, high-calorie foods turn the fatometer up, making you hungrier and hungrier.

Keeping your fatometer set as low as possible

WORTH THREE MORE STARS

Do the following to claim one star each:
- ➢ Try new foods whenever you can
- ➢ Mix up your flavours
- ➢ Have home-cooked meals whenever possible

Smart Food Choices

(Della says…)

Wow! Did you get all that about your fatometer? I must admit it took me a while to get my head around it. And even when I did, I was highly suspicious. Call me old fashioned, but I'm pretty traditional when it comes to staying slim. The thought of having a fatometer you can turn up and down in order to control your weight did take me a while to – well…um –believe!

Although once I did get my head around the science I got quite excited. Being able to control your fatometer – and we will refer to ways of doing this throughout this book – can surely only be a good thing. It can be used in combination with other methods to help you stay slim and speed up weight loss.

Now let's go on to a more traditional way of staying slim, which involves making smart food choices, but while you're making these choices, you may very well be controlling your fatometer too – which means it makes sense to bear it in mind as you read. Clever, huh!

So – what are you having for breakfast? Will you, by any chance, be taking a stroll into the canteen, or past the vending machine, and grabbing the first thing that catches your eye? It's surprising how many of us choose what we eat exactly like this. Is it wrong? No, but it might not be compatible with staying slim.

Eating loads and staying slim has a lot to do with smart food choices. If you make smart choices, you will never need to calorie count again. You will, however, need to plan what you eat. So how exactly do you make smart choices? Well, you need to know a little about food. What can you eat a lot of without taking in loads of calories (sadly it's not chocolate) and how can you cheat.

A Smart Breakfast?

(Peter says...)

Breakfast? Did somebody mention breakfast?

I love breakfast! Along with lunch and dinner it's one of my favourite meals of the day. If I had my way I'd start every day with a full English fry up. You can forget about that measly slice of toast or one of those new fangled muesli bars – they're so insubstantial I wouldn't bother feeding one to my pet hamster Eric. If I had a hamster. Called Eric or otherwise.

It will of course come as no surprise that having a substantial breakfast dramatically increases your chances of making it through to lunchtime without the need for some sort of mid-morning snack. And in my quest to find scientific, smart ways of eating I discovered that protein, rather than carbs or fat, are apparently far better at keeping the hunger pangs at bay.

So, theoretically, a protein-rich breakfast would not only be a delicious way to start the day, but should actually help you remain slender. Now if that isn't eating loads and staying slim I don't know what is.

Thing is, who has the time to start frying up fish, or a couple of steaks (or roasting pumpkin, squash or watermelon seeds) first thing in the morning? Not me. And I'm guessing not you. Which is why I created Peter's Potato & Egg Smash Up.

Peter's Potato & Egg Smash Up

Remember Basic Principle Number Seven? Of course you do. It was the one about planning. And this particular meal is a case in point. The wonderful thing about this recipe is that you'll end up with breakfast for the next four days – but you do have to do some preparation.

On Sunday (assuming you want my breakfast for Monday through to Thursday), roast some potatoes or make some chips. Now how you do this is entirely up to you but if you want to score points with Della, avoid those bags of frozen roast potatoes and make your own using the absolute minimum amount of oil. Apparently it is possible, and in a few pages' time she'll tell you how to make virtually fat free chips.

When your spuds are almost done (they're soft in the middle and beginning to turn that lovely golden brown in colour), remove them from the oven, gently break them up with the end of a rolling pin, season generously, and return to the oven.

Meanwhile take a very large wok, add a generous portion of regular olive oil (or, if your name's Della, a low fat alternative) and fry a little garlic (one or two cloves at the most – this is supposed to be breakfast), an equally small amount of chilli (maybe just one chopped green one) and a small knob of ginger. After a moment or two break eight eggs (a great source of protein) into a bowl, and add to the wok. Yes, eight eggs. Two a day for the next four days. It seems like a lot right now. Come Friday you'll wish you'd done more.

Take the potatoes out of the oven and add to the mixture. Make sure you keep turning the whole thing over with a spatula – those eggs have a habit of sticking to the bottom of the wok. Add a small handful of fresh rosemary, a glug of Worcester sauce, a small amount of soy sauce, black pepper, season a little more, and continue to cook.

When the mixture's looking 'done' (I like it fairly dry) add four teaspoons (or thereabouts) of runny honey. One teaspoon per day. Don't overdo it. True, we're creating a dish that is supposed to keep you going till lunchtime, but even so, let's at least attempt to keep the calorie count down.

Give the whole thing one last stir then transfer to a sealable plastic container, allow to cool and pop in the fridge.

Each morning use a ladle to scoop out one serving into a microwaveable bowl. Nuke it for a few seconds, then grate on a small amount of parmesan cheese (it's more protein, Della, stop looking at me like that). One quick mix with your fork – and enjoy.

Fabulous!

You might be interested to know that this particular section of the book almost never made the final draft, and that Della and I had a frank and meaningful exchange of views over whether this breakfast meets the 'stay slim' criteria of our book.

Della's argument went something like this: "You can't encourage people to use roast potatoes! They're full of fat!"

I shrugged. "It'll be OK – I'll just tell them to use your virtually fat free chip recipe or low calorie olive oil or something."

"Is that what you do?" she asked.

I recoiled in horror. "Of course not!"

"Well then!"

"Look, it's not supposed to be a fat free breakfast, it's supposed to be a high protein breakfast. It's scientifically proven that high protein -"

"There's no way that this recipe will do anything other than pack on the pounds -"

"But if it stops you from snacking…"

"Oh, don't start with that one-step-forward-two-steps-backwards thing again!"

"Plus, if it's a new flavour, then it should turn down your fatometer…"

And so the argument went on. And eventually I relented. Not because of the 'fat content' thing (personally I think fats have been unfairly demonised) but because of the carbs, and how they affect your appetite.

Whilst this is a protein-rich brekky, it's also quite high in carbohydrates which (according to some research) suppress your appetite initially, but then bring it back with a vengeance later on! This is really quite annoying. After all my efforts to come up with a delicious, high protein, hunger killing breakfast, it turns out those pesky potatoes probably neutralise the effect of the eggs.

When I admitted this to Della, she gave me one of her looks, and I took the recipe out.

Or so she thought.

Since our little spat I gave the whole protein-breakfast idea a lot of thought and came to the conclusion that if I could replace those carbs with fibre I'd have a breakfast which would muzzle my hunger for hours and hours.

A little googling later and I decided to swap the potato for *cauliflower*.

Cauliflower is high in fibre, low in carbs, and goes really well with egg. Best of all there's nothing – absolutely nothing – that Della can object to!

It tastes really good too. Give it a go.

A Smarter Breakfast

(Della says…)

I have to admit that having given Peter's breakfast section a considerable amount of thought, there are some points we both absolutely agree on. Well, one anyway.

We both love our breakfast. And it is a very important meal. A decent breakfast really will stop you feeling hungry and reaching for that mid-morning snack. Oh, I've just realised I agree with Peter on two points. But then again, I see no reason why you shouldn't reach for a mid-morning snack if you want to, as long as it's a *smart* snack (see next section).

Now then, I'm about to let you into a secret. Don't tell Peter – he's happy researching his roast potato versus cauliflower breakfast and good luck to him – however, and this may come as a surprise to some of you, it is NOT actually necessary to find an alternative to a traditional English breakfast. It is perfectly possible to start every day with a fry up. In fact, I frequently start my day with one and the only reason I don't do it more often is because I don't have the time. And yes, you can do it without putting on an ounce – or should I be talking in grams these days?

You will have to make some changes and possibly one or two compromises, but they are not onerous and they are worth it. Here's how:

✓ Remove the fat from bacon and grill instead of frying.
✓ Replace full fat meat sausages with low fat ones or low fat veggie alternatives.
✓ Fry eggs and mushrooms using a low fat spray.
✓ You might prefer to scramble or poach your eggs.
✓ Beans and tinned tomatoes are fine as they are or you could grill fresh tomatoes.

Personally, by the time I've eaten all this I don't have room for – what was it Peter said? A measly slice of toast or a new fangled muesli bar. No, I'm afraid I'm far too full!

Here are some other delicious alternatives to fry ups. Smoked haddock topped with a poached egg, or smoked salmon and scrambled eggs, are both really good fat free breakfasts. Both take under five minutes to prepare in the microwave. Fat free does not equate to taste free, particularly where breakfast is concerned, and a healthy nutritious breakfast does not take very long to prepare.

Another of my favourite breakfasts for mornings when I'd like something lighter is chopped banana and very low fat yoghurt. I happen to like very low fat yoghurt so this is a lovely breakfast for me. But you don't have to add yoghurt and don't restrict yourself to bananas. Any fresh fruit is good. Blueberries, pineapple, strawberries, raspberries, melon, prunes, mandarin segments, or perhaps a mixture of fruit salad that's been prepared the night before and left in the fridge overnight – these are all really good. There is something about fresh fruit and yoghurt that has a holiday feel about it, particularly if you use exotic fruits like lychees and figs. If you've ever been on holiday to a hotel you will probably know what I mean.

I think this is another reason I like this kind of breakfast – it has a touch of decadence about it. But don't take my word for it. Try one of these breakfasts for yourself. Try Peter's too if you like, and I hope you will bear with us on our journey through How To Eat Loads and Stay Slim. We've approached this book from entirely different angles which we hope will be helpful as well as entertaining. And yes, they can be used in combination with each other and should work. Just don't forget to check out the stars and keep an eye on your star score. And whilst we might have the odd difference of opinion we won't argue too much. I promise!

STOP! ACTION POINT!

Create a smart breakfast
(thereby reducing your need to snack)

WORTH ONE STAR FOR EACH BREAKFAST
(to a maximum of two)

Ideas you can try:

- ✓ A protein rich breakfast
- ✓ Something you can make the day (or days) before
- ✓ Fat free fry-ups
- ✓ Exotic holiday-style fruits and yogurt

Smart Snackers Stay Slim!

(Della says…)

Snacking is scrumptious, snacking is fun – and hey, if you choose smart snacks, it can help you stay slim too. There are three rules when it comes to smart snacking:

> ➤ Snacks must be fat free.
> ➤ Snacks must be within reach.
> ➤ Snacks have to be something you really, *really* want to eat.

Let's clarify that last point. Your snack has to trump everything else, i.e. you have to choose your snack as opposed to just eating it because there's nothing better on offer. Because, unless you have willpower of iron (mine's more the consistency of melted chocolate), there will always be something better.

Here are some of my favourite standby snacks – you can eat a lot of these without worrying too much about the calories.

Savoury Standby Snacks

> ➤ Hard boiled eggs. Cook a dozen at a time and put them in the fridge. They're great with salt.
> ➤ Baked beans – hot or cold.
> ➤ Prawns – with or without fat free dips.
> ➤ Poached salmon.

➢ Cold meats, such as chicken breast, turkey, ham. Or 'veggie' alternatives.

➢ Tortillas made with diced potato, ham and garlic. There are dozens of recipes available on the internet for tortillas. Just remember to use low fat spray to cook them. They are nice hot and nicer in the fridge the next day. They are also very nice with chillies if you like your food to be spicy.

➢ There are a lot of things you can make with eggs and eat cold which are fat free. Try frittatas or quiche. For quiche, substitute very low fat cottage cheese for the cream. And substitute grated potato for the pastry. This actually tastes very good. Especially when it's cold. (See our website for details.)

➢ If you really want to, and you like them, you could snack on raw vegetables, carrots, celery, peppers. But the truth is, you don't have to rely on these things.

Sweet Snacks
➢ Fat free yoghurt
➢ Fat free fromage frais
➢ Stewed apples – or any other kind of stewed fruit. (Use a sugar substitute and use cloves and ginger.) Stewed fruit is brilliant with fat free yoghurt, particularly zero per cent total fat free

yoghurt, which is the closest thing to cream I've found.

➢ Fat free jellies, particularly with fruit in them.

➢ Egg custards made with fat free fromage frais and bananas.

Snacks in the fridge

➢ Store fruit like blueberries, strawberries, grapes, melon, mango, either made up as a fruit salad with juice or alone.

➢ Fat free jellies with fruit and yoghurt – see recipe on our website.

➢ Fat free yoghurts (preferably the ones sprinkled with chocolate).

➢ Low calorie cereal bars. Anything under 100 calories. Cut them into chunks. (They take far longer to eat when they've been in the fridge).

➢ Curly Wurlys. (Yes, I did say Curly Wurlys – these are surprisingly low calorie (115 calories in a 26g size) and they take ages to eat when they've been in the fridge too.)

➢ Anything else you have prepared earlier – apple ginger clafouti, fat free cake – yes, there really is such a thing. See our website for details.

Snacks in the freezer

➢ Try frozen grapes – they're yummy. Frozen grapes are also delicious in wine.

➢ Other fruits that work well as little frozen treats are: bananas, cantaloupe (particularly nice), blueberries, fresh cherries (remove the stones first), strawberries, blackberries and clementines or any other member of the orange family.

➢ Simply slice up the fruit into bite size pieces, spread them out on a plate and pop them in the freezer for about an hour. You will be amazed at how nice frozen fruit can taste. And incidentally, bananas don't go black, which surprised me. Personally, I find frozen bananas tastier than fresh ones.

➢ Also use your freezer to stockpile sorbets – just like jacket potatoes they are a slimmer's friend.

Fat free yoghurts are great frozen, a bit like ice cream if you use your imagination (a lot!). Also, frozen yoghurts take absolutely ages to eat, which is a major advantage if you're slimming. Though perhaps I should add a word of warning here. They do get incredibly hard so go carefully. I talk from bitter experience. I have no patience whatsoever. I once tried biting into a frozen fat free yoghurt because I wanted to eat it faster than was proving to be possible.

I should have known better. I'd already bent my spoon. But not to be deterred, I picked up the whole yoghurt and bit off a chunk – at least I tried to bite off a chunk. What actually happened was that I broke off my front tooth instead. Which was extremely unpleasant, but as it happened had its own built-in slimming advantage because I couldn't eat anything at all until I got it fixed. Not, I hasten to add, that I would recommend this method of staying slim!

Oven snacks

> ➤ Baked apples – remove the cores, fill them with sultanas, a touch of cinnamon and raisins and bake. Yum.

> ➤ Baked bananas are amazing – don't remove the skins, simply slit them, insert 5 chocolate buttons and some rum if you're so inclined, although you might not fancy rum first thing in the morning! They're just as good without, don't worry. Wrap the bananas in tin foil and bake until the skins are black. (About twenty minutes in a hot oven – but check periodically.) They are delicious and work fabulously on a BBQ in the summer and they are deliciously guilt free, as long as you don't get carried away on the chocolate buttons. Top tip here is to buy small packets – not family sized ones. It's all too easy to munch your way through the rest of a family sized packet of chocolate buttons, whilst virtuously waiting for your 5 chocolate buttons in the banana to melt. I know this. I've tried it. I am not safe around chocolate buttons!

STOP! ACTION POINT!

Choose a fat free snack you really, really like!

WORTH ONE STAR FOR EACH SNACK
(to a maximum of three)

Three rules of smart snacking:

1. It must be virtually fat free.
2. It must be something you would choose over anything else.
3. It helps if you have one sweet snack and one savoury snack, so both sweet and savoury cravings are covered.

Swapping

(Della says…)

We're going to talk about substitutes a fair bit in this book. "Substitutes!" I hear you cry. "Well if you think I'm substituting chips for lettuce, forget it!" Before you fling this book across the room in disgust – wait! Hear me out. I promise I won't suggest that you swap chips for lettuce. In fact you can eat as many chips as you like, although there is one condition. You can't fry them. You will need to swap the cooking method. More about chips very shortly. But first, I would like you to consider an alternative.

Jacket Spuds

Jacket potatoes. They are an eat-loadser's best friend, providing you don't smother them in butter and cheese. You can have a small handful of cheese – and if it's a reduced fat version you can have a larger handful. But don't panic. There are plenty of other things you can smother them in. You can have beans, tuna, or any number of salad type concoctions (see Peter's 'Extreme Salads'). You can also smother them in Stir Fry, or Very Meaty Chilli, or Bolognaise (see our website for recipes), or various other tasty sauces, but you do need to swap the cooking methods and you will possibly need to use different ingredients than you usually choose. But I can promise you one thing categorically. You don't need to sacrifice taste.

The beauty of jacket potatoes is that providing you have a nice topping they're tasty, they're cheap, and you can generally get them if you're eating out, which is a bonus. They also fill you up. Don't stop at one. Have two or three if you like. I'll say it again. Jacket potatoes are an eat-loadser's best friend. They truly are.

You can also eat your potatoes steamed, boiled, mashed, roasted or fried. It is not the potato itself that is fattening; it's the fat that's used to cook it. This was a revelation for me when I learned about losing weight. A lot of the meals I really, really liked didn't have to be banned; they just had to be altered slightly to make them more slimmer friendly.

They are mostly swaps: low fat spray for oil; lean mince for regular mince; skimmed milk for full fat; half fat cheese for regular. This means that when I eat out, which I enjoy and do often, I don't have to worry too much about what I eat. I have whatever I fancy. Staying slim is about what you do *most* of the time. The odd chocolate moment or meal out is not such a heinous crime as you might think.

Here's another swap you might like:

Lasagne
I prefer my version of fat free lasagne to the full fat variety – and so do most of my foodie friends, so I know I'm not just being biased. You already know how to make a lasagne so this isn't a recipe. But it is another swap.

✓ Swap full fat mince for extra lean mince (or vegetables if vegetarian)
✓ Swap béchamel sauce for fat free fromage frais, or quark.
✓ Swap readymade sauce for canned tomatoes with basil.
✓ Swap full fat cheese for half fat cheese.

Add extra vegetables, like celery and grated carrot, regardless of whether you're making vegetarian or meat lasagne. And use herbs. They taste a lot better than fat and are a lot better for you. Try paprika, fresh basil, nutmeg, rainbow peppercorns and lemon pepper. Also, a tiny splash of very good quality balsamic works well. Vary the herbs as often as you can and you can influence your fatometer too.

Chips

I promised I'd come back to chips. You can have guilt-free chips. All you need to do is swap the method used to make them from frying to microbaking. (Microbaking, for the uninitiated, is a combination of microwave and oven baking!) You need to prepare your chips in the old fashioned way, i.e. from scratch from potatoes – frozen pre-prepared chips that you buy won't work.

Prepare the potatoes in the usual way. They don't need to be peeled – washed potatoes are fine, and probably healthier. Thick cut chips work best I find, but thin ones can be good if you're careful about cooking times.

Spread them out on a plate. Spray them with a low fat spray or use a tablespoon of olive oil. Season with salt and pepper, and microwave them for four minutes. Transfer them to the oven on a baking tray (add a little more low fat spray, if necessary) and bake at a high heat (240 C). You will need to turn them often so they get evenly browned. But this is so worth it. I promise.

You can even have tomato ketchup. You can make your own fat free tomato ketchup, but personally I don't often bother. After all, if you're saving loads of calories on the chips themselves (which you are) then why not have the real McCoy tomato sauce (whatever that means to you). For me, staying slim is about compromise. Chips made like this are not quite as good as fried chips on taste but they are totally guilt free. You can have as many as you like. They go very well with fried eggs (use low fat spray) and beans. Or ham and eggs. They also work very well if you roast vegetables alongside them (use low fat spray and black pepper). Or if you'd like cheesy chips then just sprinkle a handful of half fat grated cheese over them and melt.

And while we're on the subject of swaps, don't forget drinks.

Drink Swaps

It's so easy to watch what you eat and forget all about the liquids you put in your mouth. A friend of mine, Colin, who happens to be a chef, once told me that it's impossible to drink alcohol and eat desserts and not put on weight. You had to choose one or the other.

I suspect that Colin was right. Depending of course on what you choose to drink. In my twenties and thirties I was a 'pints of lager' girl. I only gave up my pints of lager when I joined a slimming club and realised that there was no way on earth I could fit even one pint of lager into the calorie allowance. What was I to do?

Well, actually a small glass of dry white wine isn't a bad swap for a pint of lager. Gin with slimline tonic is an even better swap. Here are some other drink swaps you might like to consider – both alcoholic drinks and other drinks.

- ✓ Swap Baileys for practically anything – and get better calorie value for your units!
- ✓ Swap beer or lager for light beer or shandy.
- ✓ Swap wine for gin or vodka.
- ✓ Swap the accompanying tonic for slimline tonic.
- ✓ Swap any soft drink, e.g. cola, ginger beer, lemonade for its low-calorie equivalent.
- ✓ Swap juice for soda water or just swap half of it for soda water.
- ✓ Swap tea with sugar and milk for tea with semi-skimmed and sweetener.

✓ Swap white tea for any herbal tea which is drunk black.

✓ Swap a smoothie for liquidised fruit with half the amount of milk (skimmed – or try half fat soya milk).

✓ Swap any sweet drink for Bovril or Marmite.

✓ Swap any drink at all for water: sparkling; still; or tap water, it doesn't matter. But do add ice and a slice.

And whatever you choose to drink that's cold, do put it in a nice glass. There are positive psychological reasons for this. You will feel as though you are getting a better deal.

More Swaps

(Peter says…)

Swapping, eh? I couldn't agree more.

For me the joy of swaps is that you're not 'cutting down' on the food or drink you like, you're merely replacing it with something similar, but better for you. There's no dieting involved. Just choices. It's all good.

Here are some swaps that have worked really well for me:

Beer

I once met a female body builder. I asked her why my abs weren't as good as hers. She prodded me in the tummy and declared that they probably were, but they were hiding under a layer of fat. Then she told me that in her experience the guys she worked out with who struggled with their weight were always beer drinkers. Knock the beer on the head, she said, and I'd lose the flab.

Easier said than done.

Especially when you're a bloke.

But it's not called a beer belly for no reason.

You could swap beer for light beer. However, in my humble opinion, as with most low fat, slimline, diet alternatives, so called light beers taste absolutely awful[2]!

---

[2] A point that Della and I have debated on more than one occasion.

But more to the point they're not as readily available in this country's pubs (which, in my mind, is no bad thing, ghastly beverages that they are).

However, here's an idea that works really well:

Swap your pints for bottles.

When your pal turns to you and asks, "What you drinking, mate?" go for a Budweiser. Or a Corona (nice with a slice of lime pushed into the neck of the bottle). Or a Becks.

Try if you can to pick something that isn't also available on draft (to avoid the possibility of getting a pint anyway). If you have a particularly generous buddy politely turn him down when he offers you two bottles. And don't ask for a glass – drink it straight from the bottle. You'll consume it slower so that it'll last roughly the same amount of time as a regular pint.

Ready to take this one step further?

Switch to wine. White wine (red wine hangovers are far worse in my experience). And learn to sip.

Now granted, there are far more calories, per ounce, in wine (especially sweet wines) than beer, but the theory is that you should consume far less. Should.

In practice I've found this only works at home in front of the telly. Or at barbecues. It never works down the pub or wherever there's a round-system in place. And it doesn't appear to work in restaurants or dinner parties either (where people have the annoying habit of refilling your glass) – before you know it you've drunk an entire bottle, perhaps more, and you're considerably more sozzled than you'd usually be had you stuck to the beer.

But it is effective.

Final word on wine. If you find your beer guzzling reflexes won't let you sip, such that you're finishing an entire bottle a night with little or no effort, try watering the wine down with at least as much soda water, preferably much more. You'll be surprised how little this impacts on the actual taste, and you'll be able to get up the following morning with no ill effects.

Crisps & Snacks
As anyone who works in a modern day office will tell you it's virtually impossible to get through the day without snacking, and during the last twenty years there have been several organisations who, at various points in their history, have struggled to keep the vending machines adequately stocked with salt & vinegar crisps. By a sheer coincidence these periods coincided with the exact moments when I was in their employ. That is, until I decided to do something about my addiction to those delightful green foil bags.

Turns out that it wasn't the actual crisps that I was addicted to, but the salt. And to a lesser or greater degree this could be satisfied by switching to those similarly sized bags of salted 'rice cakes'. Yes, true, they're not remotely cake-like, but they're still pretty tasty.

Marginally better than rice cakes was the discovery of dried fruit. Dried fruit, in my humble opinion, often tastes better than fruit. OK, not better, but less – well – fruit like, and more, you know, snack like. Which, after the 9:00am daily marketing conference call, is exactly what you need.

The problem with dried fruit is that whilst it's better for you than regular snacks (such as chocolate or crisps), gram for gram it's actually pretty high in calories. Don't go eating anything more than a small handful if you're swapping dried fruit for your mid-morning chocolate bar.

Better, in my humble opinion, than rice cakes or dried fruit are poppadums.

Poppadums[3] for those of you who aren't familiar, are the large crisp-like things they serve in Indian restaurants along with all sorts of fabulous dips. They're usually made of a non-wheat flour (such as rice or potato) and can be plain or spiced. Restaurants *used* to deep-fat-fry them (which made them slightly greasy), but it's rare for that to be the case these days.

Your average Indian supermarket[4] will sell a packet of about twenty ready-to-cook poppadums for less than

---

[3] Also known as a Papadam, pappadum, or as papad in Northern India

[4] If you don't have an Indian supermarket check the website for links to online alternatives.

a quid[5]. Look for the packets with the little Indian boy and rabbit on them. You can cook two or three poppadums in the microwave in about a minute, or under the grill (but don't take your eyes off them).

Let's consider how poppadums measure up as a potential office snack and crisp replacement. Most offices I've worked in provide a microwave in the staff kitchen. Two poppadums is a similar number of mouthfuls as your average packet of crisps, but as each poppadum is about 65 calories, you're winning by about 50 calories overall, and lowering your salt intake considerably. Result!

Sugar

As you'll probably notice, whilst Della comes at Eating Loads and Staying Slim from a traditional dieting background, I'm not in favour of any food products that have the words light, low fat, or slimline printed on them. I like butter! I like cheese! And I like sugar in my tea! I like food to taste nice – the 'diet' versions of most foods seem to achieve their godly status by losing the very element that made me want to eat them in the first place – flavour.

Nowhere is this more evident than with sugar. I've tried numerous different artificial sweeteners over the

---

[5] Your average mainstream super market will sell packets of half a dozen, ready-to-eat poppadums for a small fortune. In my humble opinion these are nowhere near as good and I have no idea how they measure up, calorie wise.

years (which I can't mention here because I don't want to have to defend my comments in court) and without exception they all taste hideous!

You could try natural alternatives. For instance, I use honey in camomile tea and occasionally in coffee, though it does have a flavour of its own, and it's also packed with calories[6].

When it comes to swapping sugar, it seems that there just isn't a low fat, healthier alternative that doesn't alter the taste beyond acceptable levels.

The curious thing about sugar, however, is that it's a little like gangster rap music. It doesn't matter how quietly you play your gangster rap music, it's always loud. You can turn it down and my ears will register that there's slightly less volume, but if I can still hear it, it's still loud (and I'd really like you to turn it off).

Likewise, sugar is a 'loud' flavour. It doesn't really matter how much is in your food, or in your tea or coffee, you can always taste it. Sure, if you add more, or take some away, your taste buds recognise the fact, but it's still there. It's a 'loud' flavour.

What's more, just like gangster rap music, I can only tell whether there's more or less sugar based on how much there was previously.

Which, being a total nerd, I find utterly fascinating.

---

[6] Interestingly, whilst researching this section I found a suggestion that cinnamon might work as an alternative to sugar. I'll try it out and report back.

The swap for sugar – so I've discovered – is actually 'less sugar'. And to get around that unpleasant sensation of noticing that there is 'less', the trick is to reduce the amount of sugar you use very, very gradually. And the only way to do that is to measure it accurately.

Take tea, for instance. For much of my life I was a two heaped teaspoons of sugar kinda guy. And as I drank maybe seven or eight cups of tea a day, that's quite a lot of sugar. In fact, assuming that each teaspoon of sugar is 4 grams, and that a gram of sugar is 3.8 calories, it's an extra thirty calories a cup, and two hundred and forty-three calories a day[7]. Which is pretty meaningless to non-dieters such as myself, but it must be a lot because Jules (my assistant – a two sugars in her tea lady) went extremely pale when I told her.

Anyway, to swap 'sugar' with 'less sugar' I obtained a set of measuring spoons (very cheap, available online or from any store that sells kitchenware) and placed them into the sugar bowl. Every time I made a cuppa, I diligently measured out the sugar properly (it honestly took longer to type that sentence than it takes in real life). Over a period of several *weeks* (days won't work) I gradually went from two teaspoons to a quarter of a teaspoon – which is what I have today. The tea still tastes sweet, but I've reduced my sugar intake by almost ninety per cent. And the tiny little 'quarter of a teaspoon'

---

[7] One thousand seven hundred ish a week. Whilst we're crunching numbers.

spoon that still sits in the bowl is a reminder as to what I achieved.

Go ahead. Roll your eyes. But it works, and it's definitely worth a try.

(Della says...)
Sorry to butt in here, folks, but if you were rolling your eyes – ahem – at this cutting down sugar method mooted by my esteemed co-author, then you might want to take a quick peek at my section, Acquiring Good Taste. My cutting out sugar method might just work better for you! Please do feel free to leave a comment on our website about which method works the best – not that I'm trying to be competitive here, much!

Shop Bought Burgers
(Peter says...)
Whilst I'm baring my soul with my fondness for sugar, beer and crisps I might as well go the whole hog and talk about burgers. (I can feel Della shaking her head in despair.)

When I was a kid beef burgers were a forbidden food. My mother suspected that they, along with sausages and pork pies, were made of parts of the animal you wouldn't eat even if someone offered you hard cash to do so. However, their prohibited status made them far more attractive and as a result I developed a love for all three, which has lasted my entire life.

I'm not even talking about home-made burgers from prime cut beef that you've minced yourself and carefully moulded into patties; I'm talking about shop bought frozen burgers, the ones you throw under the grill when you can't be bothered to do real cooking.

Imagine my total and utter shock then when I discovered that most veggie alternatives *actually taste better*.

I don't expect you to believe me. Honestly, I don't. Because I've been where you are and I wouldn't have believed me either. So instead I want to set you a challenge.

Buy a small packet of veggie burgers, and try one. Treat it exactly as you would do a normal burger.

The first thing you'll notice is that it's silent. There aren't those satisfying pop and sizzle sounds that burgers usually make as the fat ignites. Second thing you'll notice is the absence of that lovely burger smell. But once you've melted some cheese on top and put it between two halves of a burger bun, with some lettuce, sliced onion, mustard and ketchup, a rather amazing thing happens.

It looks exactly like a burger.

And dependent on the brand of veggie burger it'll either taste like one – I mean, *indistinguishable* – or better! Apart from being less greasy, of course. And wait, there's something else missing – how come I haven't chipped a tooth on anything that looks suspiciously like gristle yet? Because there isn't any!

Let's leave it there. I've got more to say on the subject of veggie food but that's a topic for another chapter. For the moment if you have any suggestions for food swaps, visit the website[8], click the 'swaps' category over on the right, and share them with the world in the comments section.

[8] www.howtoeatloadsandstayslim.com

STOP! ACTION POINT!

Swapping

ONE STAR FOR EACH SWAP
(to a maximum of five stars)

Flick back through the previous pages and see if there are any foods you could painlessly swap for healthier, less fattening alternatives – at least some of the time.
Pay particular attention to:

- ➢ chips for jacket spuds
- ➢ all manner of alcoholic beverages for other equally alcoholic, less horrific, less calorific alternatives
- ➢ Sugar for less sugar (with the aid of measuring spoons)
- ➢ Crisps, burgers and snack foods for healthier and shockingly tasty alternatives

Planning

(Della says...)

Swapping will require some forward planning. You will need to make sure you have these healthy swaps available at all times, or the ingredients to make them. Until meal planning becomes second nature to you, this is probably the hardest bit to do. When I first started doing it, I realised that what I actually needed to do was to introduce another stage to my shopping expeditions.

The extra stage involved deciding what I was going to eat that was low fat and tasty, and then making sure I had the ingredients. Often I would be missing ingredients like herbs – which weren't in big demand for my ready-meal style brand of cooking.

After all, we all have to go shopping; it's one of those tedious little facts of life. What we buy while we're there is up to us.

So, decide what you are going to eat. Make a list and go shopping. By the way, one of my top tips for shopping is never to attempt it on an empty stomach. It's much easier to buy only the items on your list if you're not starving. Shop with your head, not your stomach!

So, just to kick things off, why don't we have a go at that right now while I'm here? No, I am not going to come shopping with you – I have my own to do – but maybe I can help with the planning side of things.

Plan Three Meals

Yes, I know there are more than three days in a week, but let's not get carried away. You can always do another plan later.

Do the following:

➢ Decide on three lunches. Frittata and fat free quiche are transportable and tasty. There are recipes for both on our website.

➢ Decide on three main meals. They may not be that different from what you usually have. A cottage pie, a lasagne or a stew are fine; just use extra lean meat and don't add fat. But do add a vegetable you've never tried before – chopped celery's good in all of the above, and so is grated carrot. See our website for more inspiration.

➢ If you need dessert – and let's face it, who doesn't? – then make one. You'll need to swap sweetener for sugar, fromage frais or quark for cream. I recommend my apple ginger clafouti – recipe on our website.

➢ Make a list of all the ingredients you need.

➢ Go shopping.

➢ Cook.

➢ Enjoy!

> **STOP! ACTION POINT!**
>
> Plan (and execute) three meals
>
> TWO STARS FOR EACH
> (so six in total)

Final thoughts
- ➢ You'll probably have to go shopping more often.
- ➢ You will have to cook.
- ➢ I didn't say it was going to be easy!

This Chapter is NOT About Vegetables

(Peter says…)

I love vegetables.

Let me say that again.

I love vegetables.

Notice how effortlessly I put those words on the page – how easily they flow from my head, through my fingers, before appearing before your eyes.

I love vegetables.

Aren't you impressed? No? It's taken me over forty years to get to the point where I can say that. But I swear to you it's the God's honest truth, and by now I'm sure you realise that I'm a man of my word.

Apart from when it came to putting a title on this chapter.

Sorry about that.

Vegetables Are Boring

(Peter says...)

For most of my life vegetables were 'evil'.

I blame my mother.

As a child, most of my meals were of the 'meat and two veg' variety and when (as a lot of kids do) I turned my nose up at what she'd slaved over, she told me to "at least eat the meat".

Also, she let me leave home. That was pretty much the death knell in my relationship with anything green. I finally had a chance to eat the food that I liked. Which basically amounted to pizza.

Or burgers.

Or ready meals.

When I did finally attempt to cook something as adventurous as, say, a roast chicken, other than potatoes I skimped out on the veggies completely. They just weren't interesting enough. They were, on the whole, pretty darn boring.

And that's a problem.

Because they also happen to be really good for you.

You've probably heard it said that you should eat five portions of fruit or vegetables per day. There's a reason for that. Vegetables are absolutely stuffed full of goodness. More interestingly though, they even contain some of the nutrients that some would have you believe only come from meat or dairy products – such as protein, or calcium! Who knew?! (Well obviously lots of smart people, but I wasn't one of them.)

From an eat-loadser's point of view vegetables are also at the top of the leader board.

The vast majority of veg contain less than a gram of fat per serving, and the fats they do contain are usually *un*saturated (that's the good kind). More than that, many vegetables take almost as many calories to eat and digest than you ultimately get from them. Meaning that there are very few excess calories to be stored as fat. And because vegetables are high in fibre you feel fuller, faster – all of which means you'd really have to go some to put on weight *if* your meals consisted of nothing but vegetables.

Now don't panic – I'm not going to tell you that meat is *bad* for you (protein, as you know, fills you up for longer) – but the fact is that less meat on your plate, and more veg, would pretty much guarantee a slimmer you in the long term. If you can break your reliance on meat you'll be one huge step towards being able to eats loads, and stay slim, forever. Which would be very good news – if only vegetables weren't so blinkin'…

BORING!!!

I genuinely believe the *real* reason more people aren't vegetarian or vegan is that, compared to a stick of celery or a serving of carrots, a great fat juicy steak, pan-fried in butter, just *tastes* better.

And therein is the solution to our problem. If vegetables fill you up, and give you loads of nutrients, all without letting you pile on the pounds, we simply need to find a way to make them more interesting to our palates.

How to Make Vegetables Taste Better

(Peter says…)

Here's a thing that only occurred to me a year or so ago, and something you may not have considered before:

VEGETABLES
ARE NOT
ELECTRIC GUITARS

Well of course not. But what I mean is there isn't anything remotely rock 'n' roll about vegetables.

Meat, on the other hand…

A home-made burger of freshly ground beef, topped with melted cheese, between two bits of home-made crusty bread, is like a four piece rock band, turning your taste buds into screaming adoring fans. Meat is very rock 'n' roll. And what occurred to me, after twenty something years of preparing my own meals, is that every time I tried to get a vegetable onto my plate I treated it the same as the meat. The food equivalent of introducing a clarinet player into my imaginary rock band.

But vegetables aren't electric guitars.

They're orchestral.

Five or six years ago now I met my friend and fellow author Wendy Steele. Wendy is a wheat and dairy intolerant vegetarian so you can imagine how slender she is. You might also assume – wrongly – that cooking for her would be a bit of a nightmare. That's OK. I did too. For the first few months of our friendship, if Wendy came over for the day she'd bring a packed lunch because I wouldn't know what to prepare for her.

Then one day she rocked up with a carrier bag of carrots, leeks, onions, garlic, broad beans, cabbage, mushrooms, broccoli, a handful of herbs and a bag of brown rice, and suggested that we make something together. I dug around in a cupboard, found a wok that until then had never been used, and twenty minutes later I was tucking into the biggest vegetarian stir fry I'd ever had. Actually, let me clarify that – it was the *only* vegetarian stir fry I'd ever had.

And it was fabulous.

Even as I type this now my stomach is rumbling at the very thought of it. On that day I started to discover the simple secret to enjoying vegetables:

COMBINE AS MANY AS POSSIBLE

Whoever came up with the "eat five portions of fruit and veg a day" advice neglected to mention that it's actually easier to do this, and far tastier, if all five portions are in the same meal.

Vegetables, like instruments in an orchestra, are better in abundance. The more instruments you have in an orchestra, the richer the sound – the more vegetables you mix together whilst creating a meal, the better they taste.

And just as not all instruments are created equal in the sound department, there are certain vegetables that pack more punch in the flavour department. Garlic, chilli and ginger are always an excellent way to start any stir fry or vegetarian dish.

If you don't fancy stir frying your veg, then roast them. Vegetables respond really well to roasting.

Try this:

Peter's Veggie Bake

Take the largest roasting dish you have, and grease with butter or oil. Slice a potato or two (no more) – or a turnip, or three or four parsnips – and lay the slices on the bottom of the dish. Take as many vegetables as you can (carrots, broccoli, cauliflower, aubergine, leeks – whatever you can find), chop them up and layer them. Don't forget several cloves of (roughly chopped) garlic, and maybe some ginger. Drizzle a little more oil on the veg. Remember to season. Then pour on a white/cheese sauce. Don't buy a sauce, make your own: Take a pint of (semi) skimmed milk (cow's milk or an alternative), add a knob (just a knob) of butter, and warm slowly, adding a couple of teaspoons of cornflour every thirty seconds and whisking continuously. When the mixture begins to stiffen take off the heat immediately. Add a handful of grated cheddar cheese (just the one handful) then pour onto your veggies.

Top the whole thing with breadcrumbs. Again don't buy them. Save bits of old bread in the freezer, and grind them to crumbs in the food processor. Cover the whole thing with foil (shiny side down). Bake for an hour and a half at around 170 degrees Celsius (Gas mark 3). The longer you bake the better it gets – just try not to burn the top.

Cut into portions and serve one slice (per person) with a little ketchup or chilli sauce. If it looks lonely on the plate, amazingly it goes really really well with a side salad (don't groan – it works). Put the rest in the fridge; it will taste even better tomorrow (honest – you'll be surprised). Reheat it in the oven for five or ten minutes when you're ready to eat. Whatever you have left over after tomorrow can be frozen (thaw before reheating).

Now it's going to come as no surprise to some of you that my esteemed co-author almost had heart failure when she saw the list of ingredients: butter, oil, cheese, breadcrumbs… It was almost enough to put her off her fat free dessert (though not enough to prevent her from clearing the plate when I made this dish for her), and for the second time in this book one of my recipes was called into question. To which I offer the following defence:

Firstly, the point here is not to create a fat free meal, but to help you break your reliance on meat and convenience foods, and re-introduce you to vegetables which are, by their very nature, very low in fats, fabulously good for you, and lip-smackingly delicious… if you use plenty of them.

Secondly, if you're truly worried about the calorie count I encourage you to use Della's fat free cooking principles to turn this dish into a slightly more wholesome, guilt-free version.

By the way, this recipe is even better if you throw in some fresh herbs: sage, rosemary, thyme etc. These herbs grow really well – in pots or in the ground – all year round in the British climate, so save yourself some money and start growing your very own vegetable enhancers.

Della's got more to say on the subject of herbs and spices, but before she grabs back control of the book, let's tackle those salads.

Salads

(Peter says...)

When it comes to salads, the same rule applies. Get as many different things on your plate as possible, and mix them up.

When I was a kid a salad consisted of the following:

- ✓ iceberg lettuce
- ✓ sliced tomato
- ✓ sliced cucumber
- ✓ grated carrot
- ✓ ham

...each occupying its own section of the plate.

That is not a salad.

Try this:

Peter's Extreme Salad

Toast ONE slice (per person) of granary[9] bread[10] and then cut into small cubes – like croutons, except that these haven't been fried. Sprinkle half on the bottom of

---

[9] If you only have white bread, skip this step and throw that white loaf out for the birds and never buy it again. There's nothing fine about those refined flours – they're bad for you. They're not good for the birds either, but there are more of them than there are of you.

[10] By the way, Della recoils in horror at the thought of using bread in a salad. She says bread is fattening. Pffff! OK, it probably is – but you're making a salad and breaking your reliance on meat – it's a huge step in the right direction. I think you can be forgiven for one slice of bread! I won't tell her if you won't.

a dish. Next take your lettuce (not iceberg – iceberg must be the most tasteless lettuce on the planet. There are a million different varieties. Try rocket, cos, spinach, basil, thinly sliced cabbage, all of the above…) and lay over the top. Then add some tomato. Slice some cucumber. Scrape out the seeds and the white bits from a chilli, chop the rest finely, and sprinkle on top. Add some red onion. Or pickled silverskin onions. Sweetcorn. Red peppers (for colour). Season (that's important). Top with the remaining 'non-croutons'. Then – very very important – drizzle generously with extra virgin olive oil (no low fat alternatives please), and a few splashes of balsamic vinegar. Wow! Now that's a salad.

But wait – feeling really hungry? Need warming up a bit? Boil some small new potatoes, pile those in the middle, put a dollop (just a dollop) of (garlic) mayo[11] on top. The whole thing shouldn't take you much more than fifteen minutes (regardless of how many people you're feeding).

I called this an 'extreme salad'. It's one of my favourite meals – tastes better and better as you work your way through it – and always goes down well with guests.

---

[11] So long as you're only putting a tablespoon-sized dollop on go ahead and use the full fat stuff.

And if you only knew how much my stomach is rumbling! So whilst I go and make some lunch, time for you to do some work.

Give vegetables a chance

WORTH ONE STAR FOR TRYING,
SEVEN STARS IF YOU TURN SEMI-VEGGIE

Commit to creating at least one meal this week that's pretty much vegetarian/vegan. If it goes well, commit to another.

Do the following:
> Work as many vegetables into the meal as possible. At least six different kinds on your plate. Mix them up!
> Put aside all thoughts like "I don't like onions" or "I don't like broccoli" – when combined with other ingredients they'll taste completely different.
> Use garlic, ginger or chilli. Maybe all three.
> Use herbs.
> Season.

Final thoughts

> Other than potatoes do not boil your veg (unless you're making soup). Boiling removes nutrients, and flavour. Use a steamer or microwave.

> The aim here *isn't* to create a fat free meal – that's a by-product. We're merely trying to break your reliance on meat and/or processed convenience foods.

Herbs And Hot Stuff

(Della says…)

I like strong flavours. I like my food to be interesting. Taste is everything to me.

When it comes to flavour, a lot of popular meals rely on fats, because fats taste good. Fat combines well with sugars and grains and therefore is the main ingredient in a lot of calorie-laden desserts and sauces. It also helps to make meats moist and tender.

Fat is, however, nine calories per gram, so low calorie meals tend to rely on the fat being removed. An unfortunate consequence of this is loss of flavour.

However, the really good news is that you do not need to ever eat bland food again. Herbs and spices also add flavour to food. Varying the taste of your food will also help to lower your fatometer. And I can't think of a single herb or spice that isn't fat free. Use your imagination. But here are a few of my favourite herbs and spice food combos:

Savoury stuff
- ➢ Beef – smoked paprika, ginger
- ➢ Chicken – garlic, sage, cumin, lemongrass (maybe not all at once!)
- ➢ Stir fry – Chinese five-spice
- ➢ Tomatoes – fresh basil and black pepper
- ➢ Cheese – lemon pepper
- ➢ Hard boiled eggs – paprika

- Savoury rice – saffron
- Jacket potatoes – rainbow pepper

Sweet stuff
- Plain yoghurt – cinnamon,
- Stewed fruit – ginger, cloves, cinnamon

Also, try perking up your food with soy sauce, good quality balsamic vinegar, fish sauce, teriyaki, lemon juice, honey. Experiment – don't be worried about making mistakes. I'm lucky enough to have three dogs who are quite keen on my mistakes. Not a lot gets wasted in our house

Hot stuff
Chillies deserve a special mention. As well as perking up your food no end, chillies are fat free. But there is one other very good reason to eat them. There is quite a bit of evidence to suggest that they can speed up weight loss.

This is because they contain a chemical called capsaicin. Capsaicin is thought to help speed up your metabolism and also to oxidise fat. Incidentally, it is also found in the non-hot variety of peppers such as cayenne peppers (red peppers), which is handy if you're not keen on chillies. If you don't like peppers at all, you can buy cayenne supplements from health food shops.

For as long as I can remember I've had a love affair with chillies – the hotter they are, the more I like them.

This is probably because I was brought up in a house where we always had language students, many of whom were fond of cooking. So while other kids in my road were tucking into fish and chips or ham and tomato omelettes, we were eating chilli con carnies. I've been a fan of chillies ever since.

Blowing Hot and Cold

Chillies are brilliant in salads. They add flavour as well as heat. I slice them up very thinly and scatter them over my leaves, sweetcorn, onions, cucumber, a few olives and capers. You might want to remove the seeds, I don't bother. I like my meals hot.

If you use fresh chillies, though, check the heat levels. They vary hugely. In the past I've grown my own and I've noticed that there can be a big difference in strength, even from the same plant. I know people who wear gloves to handle them. I don't do this, but I do wash my hands with soap – water by itself isn't enough – after handling chillies. Accidentally transferring a seed to your eye is no fun at all.

Chopped fresh chillies are a good way to spice up home-made quiches and frittatas. They also go well in omelettes – try chilli and anchovy together, that works well. They are a good addition (in moderation if you don't like your food too spicy) to prawn and chicken pasta dishes, and they are also a very good barbecue ingredient. If you make home-made beef burgers, and would like to spice them up, add chillies. You'll never be accused of serving bland burgers again. They're good for adding to fish on the BBQ too. Chop them finely and add to fresh tuna or salmon with lemon juice and ginger.

STOP! ACTION POINT!

Herbs and hot stuff

WORTH ONE STAR FOR TRYING,
AND ANOTHER IF YOU STICK TO IT

Try any of the following:
- ➢ Work some of the herbs/spices mentioned in this section into your meals, both sweet and savoury
- ➢ Buy a bottle of chilli sauce, or a pot of crushed chillies

Surviving Social Eating

(Della says…)

For most of us, eating is part of our social lives and, even if it isn't, we rarely eat alone. When you embark on a weight loss campaign, do you go through your diary and delete all engagements that involve eating out or eating with other people? If so, then this is a "must read" section for you. Plus, I have some very good news.

You do not have to dine alone. You can eat out, attend dinner parties and cook meals for your family. All you have to do is cheat a little.

How To Cheat Your Dinner Guests

If I'm trying to lose weight then dinner parties are out – true? Not necessarily. Your host may well be serving food that falls into your smart food choices anyway. If they are not, then don't worry. Like any other type of social occasion that involves eating, the odd one won't hurt you. You can eat out regularly too as long as you make smart choices.

But first, let's start with dinner parties where you're in control of the cooking. These are the simplest. Cook your guests a cordon bleu meal they'll never forget.

Here's a sample menu:

DELLA'S SAMPLE MENU

Vegetable roulade with a mint dressing
(One pea on a plate with a smidgeon of mint sauce)
***

Grilled salmon
(as it sounds – small piece, skin removed)
***

Fresh fruit with coulis
(one strawberry, sliced, and one mashed)
***

Coffee with mint
(mint leaf, that is!)

I am joking, of course. Well, actually, I wasn't joking about one thing. If you serve up this meal to your guests, I doubt very much they will ever forget it. Maybe if you don't like them very much and would prefer them not to come back for a repeat performance, it might be worth it.

No, really, I am joking. But hang on a minute, there is an element of truth behind every joke. Don't discard my sample menu too hastily. After all, it was fat free, wasn't it? You could eat it and stay slim, couldn't you? You could eat it and lose a lot of weight – if not actually starve to death!

There's a lot to be said for cordon bleu, if you don't mind stopping for fish and chips on the way home (which is what my family do if we're ever invited to this type of meal). But this book is, after all, about eating loads and staying slim.

So what if we were to make a few additions? Let's have another look at that menu:

DELLA'S MUCH BETTER SAMPLE MENU

Scallops with ginger, chilli and spring onion on a mint
pea puree
(Yum)
***

Grilled salmon with asparagus, green beans,
sweetcorn and baby new potatoes
(quite yum too if you're into fish)
***

Baked bananas with a raspberry coulis
(make coulis with sweetener, not sugar)
***

Coffee with mint
(Go on, have a chocolate one,
it's the only fattening bit of the menu!)

You might also want to swap the salmon for steak, if you'd prefer a less fishy menu, and swap the new potatoes for potato wedges (use a low fat spray) or a potato and onion rosti or dauphinoise made with fat free fromage frais. You could also have a sorbet between courses if you want to be posh!

The beauty of dinner parties is that your guests won't want to feel over full. Taste is more important. So they are actually not as lethal for your waistline as you might think and if you're going to cook anyway, then you may as well cook fat free healthy food.

How To Cheat Your Spouse

(Della says…)

This will, of course, depend on your spouse. If they're the sort of person who likes to 'help out' in the kitchen then it's trickier. I recommend barring them – say you're cooking a surprise meal or doing something new you need to concentrate on – particularly if he/she is traditional about food and will object to you using some new fangled ingredient (like semi skimmed milk!).

Basically with spouses and children what the eye doesn't see the taste buds are unlikely to object to. At least, this is the case in our house. It is the thought of me using a low fat spray, or a reduced fat cheese or, heaven forbid, some vegetarian ingredient like soya that my husband doesn't like. If he doesn't see what I am up to in the kitchen he is perfectly happy.

In fact, when I decided I wanted to stay permanently slim, and became interested in cooking healthier recipes, making a very low fat version of our favourite meals without him noticing became something of a personal challenge. We also argued about it, although not in the way you might expect.

I'd cook meals he thought were delicious, for example beef stew (not that I'm one for blowing my own trumpet, you understand). He'd say, 'I bet this isn't fat free.'

I'd say, 'It is actually,' and he wouldn't believe me. 'No way!'

'Yes way!'

'Really?!'

'Really, honestly, it's fat free. Well, virtually fat free.'

Technically, when I lost weight he should have lost it too – but he would usually make up for any calorific advantages by eating chocolate in front of the telly. I have not managed to find a fat free substitute for chocolate. If anyone else has got one, please do email me with details (as soon as possible!)

How To Cheat Your Children

(Della says…)

I think this is harder than 'cheating' your spouse or your dinner party guests. But for once in this book I'm going to be serious and say that perhaps it's best not to bother even trying. Perhaps it's best just to tell them the truth. Because despite all my flippancy, I do actually care passionately about food and healthy eating and I know from experience how wonderful it is to lose weight without pain, to eat lovely food without guilt, and to fit into my clothes without starving myself. And it is so much easier to do all of these things when you know about food – and you know how to make healthy choices.

So forgive me for being serious for a moment but I think that the very best thing we can do for our children is to get them involved and to teach them how to cook with healthy ingredients. Because their future health and happiness, and possibly their self esteem too, depends on it. And isn't that the best gift we can possibly give them?

My grandmother taught me to cook. I have the best, best memories of standing on a chair in her kitchen, getting covered in flour and learning how to make mince pies and flapjacks and cakes. I don't think we ever made a fat free dish in our lives.

With one exception – stewed apples. The apples came straight from the trees in her garden. She would have hated to see me using sweetener instead of sugar, though! It was Gran who taught me to always use the same amount of cloves – four – so you knew exactly how many to hook out later on before you ate them.

When Gran passed away I inherited her cooking scales (still in their ancient box), her orange squeezer, her hard boiled egg slicer, her silver cutlery and a host of other much loved, much used implements.

Whenever I cook I feel as though Gran is beside me – but I don't cook many of her recipes, except at Christmas when I don't care if I pile on the pounds – because I've yet to find a way to make fat free pastry. (If you have found one – then same rules as for the chocolate substitute – please email it to me NOW.) Not very many of my gran's recipes can be converted to fat free.

And that's quite sad, isn't it?

Wouldn't it be good if we could give our children a way of cooking that they can use forever? A way of cooking that is healthy and good for them? What a legacy that would be.

Eating Out – How To Make Smarter Choices

(Della says…)

I love eating out. And it is perfectly possible for an eat-loadser to dine out regularly and still stay slim (or lose weight if that's your preference). But you need to make smart choices. And you also need enough confidence to ask for what you want. If it's not on the menu that doesn't mean it isn't available.

I don't mean you should change every item on the menu, just for fun, but you can ask for small changes – don't be afraid to ask how food is prepared either, i.e. is it fried, grilled, or baked?

But let's start at the beginning.

Smart Choice – Starters

Melon is an excellent choice. It's fat free; it's one of your five a day. It's a bit boring though, isn't it? I never choose melon. Most things are more interesting than melon.

Soups can be good for slimmers – they can also be very, very bad. Generally speaking, clear soups, like French onion, or tomato based soups or vegetable based soups are great. Cream based soups or ones with rich cheeses like stilton are not so great. Watch out for croutons which tend to be fried. Also, soups tend to be served with hunks of bread and butter. Great hunks of bread and butter are never going to be a smart choice.

You could try handing them immediately to your dining partner – unless they're an eat-loadser too – or you could ask for them not to be served in the first place. I know from experience that it's much more difficult to resist something once it has been put in front of you.

Prawns and all things fishy – for example, smoked trout, mackerel, smoked salmon etc. – are a good choice too. Avoid accompanying sauces. And avoid fish if it's made into paté.

Smart Choice – Mains
Generally speaking, fish is good as a main course too – especially when it's baked, or grilled. The main exception to this rule is when it's covered in batter (sadly), or when it's swimming in a creamy sauce or butter sauce. If fish does come with a creamy sauce and you really can't bear to have it without, then ask for the sauce to come separately in a jug. Restaurants are usually happy to oblige. This does not mean you can then pour the whole jug on, by the way; it means you can be more sensible – you can do your own portion control.

If you are unable to be sensible that day (I occasionally fall into this category) then don't get the jug. The jug is an option for sensible diners.

Better still, go for a tomato based sauce. Tomato based sauces – like jacket potatoes – are an eat-loadser's best friend. And you can have as much of them as you like.

The vegetables in restaurants often come separately – and they are often presented dripping in butter. When you order your food, ask for the butter to be left off. "But I like butter," I hear you say. Well, that may be the case, but trust me, you'll get used to vegetables without it. They actually taste better without it after a while. Try pepper!

Chicken, when it's not fried, is generally a good choice. New potatoes or jackets are better than any other kind of potatoes. No butter – sorry.

Omelettes or frittatas or stir fries are a good choice. Pies or roast dinners or chips or anything with creamy sauces are not. Mixed grills aren't a bad choice – but watch out if they come with chips – and of course they are often fried and not grilled at all. Ask if you're not sure.

Smart Choice – Salads

Salads – ah yes, salads. Now, you do not need to eat salads to stay slim, as we've already discussed. But if you like salads then they can be a very good choice in restaurants.

Choose tuna or prawn or chicken or meat salads – but be careful if they come smothered in creamy dressings (you can ask for these to be left off or to come separately) and go easy on cheese salads. Top choices would probably be grilled chicken, salmon or prawn.

Personally, I find that salads tend to be a little unadventurous in most restaurants (I've yet to find a local one that uses chillies, for example), and one of the reasons I like salads at home is because I can put my own dressing on them.

Restaurants will often provide a fat free dressing if you ask. But there is nothing to stop you taking your own. I often take my own. See our website for how to make it. Then I surreptitiously pour it on when no one is looking. I put it in a small plastic tub and also a sealed plastic bag. Don't forget the plastic bag if it's going in your handbag. If you're a man reading this, then I'm not sure where you're going to put it. Maybe Peter can answer that one!

Smart Choice – Desserts

Now, on to desserts. These are probably the trickiest part of a meal in a restaurant. It is hard to find a good, smart choice dessert: hard, but not impossible.

Fruit salads and sorbets are good choices. If there is baked fruit, that's a good choice too. Meringues are possible. Ice cream isn't that bad. Worst choices in restaurants are likely to be pies, crumbles, cheesecakes and cake-style puddings – oh, and anything creamy. Cheese and biscuits are quite a bad choice too, unfortunately.

If you really want a calorie-laden dessert, then my advice is to have it, but compromise on something else. Perhaps you could have a dessert instead of wine.

I tend to relax when I'm eating out. I don't worry too much about it as I use healthy cooking principles at home. And I don't eat out more than once a week. But I do make deals with myself, such as I'll have an ultra smart main course and no wine and then I'll have dessert. Or I'll have a slightly naughtier main course but no dessert. I'll save myself for the fat free scrummy dessert I have in my fridge at home.

This last option is not as hard as you might think. Chances are you'll be too full at the restaurant anyway. It'll also be cheaper!

And if you are anything like me, you will be able to cope with temporary denial, as long as you know you can have something lovely and sweet later. Waiting for a treat is possible. Knowing I can never have a treat is not!

Incidentally, if I know I'm going somewhere – a party, for instance, or even just to meet a group of friends – where there will be no fat free treats available and where they will be eating cakes, then I do take my own healthy treats (and I don't mean apples). This way, I can join in. I can still be part of the group. I don't feel as though I'm missing out.

This only works, by the way, if it's a treat you really enjoy. I did try taking apples once, but it didn't work because I didn't really want to eat apples. I wanted to eat cake.

So these days, I make my own fat free cakes. See the recipe on our website.

Smart Choice – Coffee

Don't get caught out at this late stage of the meal. Coffee is often served with a jug of cream. And it's all too easy to pour it in without a thought.

Ask for semi-skimmed milk instead. Or you could drink it black. If it's good coffee it's often nicer black. Oh, and by the way it is not compulsory to eat the mint/biscuit/chocolate etc. that comes with the coffee.

Although actually if it's a home-made chocolate – that would be at a special meal, probably – then I have to confess I can't resist.

A good question to ask yourself – in any situation where you need to make a choice – might be:

IS IT WORTH THE CALORIES?

If it is, then have it. And let's face it, you won't always know until you try it. But quite often food is not worth the calories. If, for example, I know that a restaurant where I go does not do yummy home-made desserts but serves up a thin piece of insipid cheesecake that has only just thawed out, then I might make a decision that it's really not worth the calories. And wait until I get home. Or if it does do home-made desserts I might actually have a light lunch so I can fit one in!

Before I leave this section, I really should mention the kind of restaurants which are traditionally more dangerous for eat-loadsers. Here is a quick guide to some of the smart choices there. This section is also relevant to takeaways.

Indian Restaurants

Best Choice:
- ➤ Oven baked tandoori dishes, tikka dishes
- ➤ Plain boiled rice or basmati rice
- ➤ Many sizzling dishes

Worst Choice:
- ➤ Cream based curries (masalas)
- ➤ Rich curries (madras etc)
- ➤ Naan bread

Chinese Restaurants

Best Choice:
- ➤ Noodles with chicken, vegetables, beef
- ➤ Stir fry dishes
- ➤ Prawn chow mein
- ➤ Chop suey

Worst Choice:
- ➤ Curries
- ➤ Anything in batter
- ➤ Fried rice
- ➤ Sweet and sour sauces

NB: Try using chopsticks where appropriate. They are a great slimming aid. Particularly if you're not very good with them! Don't restrict their use to Chinese takeaways – try them with other kinds of meals. Taking a long time to eat your food gives your brain the time to register that your stomach is full.

Italian Restaurants
Best Choice:
- ➤ Tomato based pastas, chicken, shellfish
- ➤ Risottos are fine if not creamy
- ➤ Salads

Worst Choice:
- ➤ Pizzas
- ➤ Pastas with creamy sauces
- ➤ Garlic breads or bruschetta

Thai Restaurants
Best Choice:
- ➤ Noodles with meat or veg
- ➤ Clear soups
- ➤ Vegetable mixes
- ➤ Fish
- ➤ Chicken
- ➤ Satays

Worst Choice:
- ➤ Rich creamy sauces
- ➤ Coconut milk based sauces
- ➤ Peanut dishes

➢ Spring rolls

Japanese Restaurants

Best Choice:
➢ Sushi
➢ Fish
➢ Soya
➢ Tofu
➢ Lean meat
➢ Brown rice
➢ Anything steamed or grilled

Worst Choice:
➢ Sticky rice
➢ Some bean curd recipes
➢ Anko (made of beans and sugar)
➢ Fried dumplings
➢ Tempura

Fish and Chip Restaurants

Best Choice:
➢ Erm – I have to confess fish and chip restaurants are tricky. Would you be content with a carton of mushy peas? No? Then maybe traditional fish and chip shops are not the best place to go. Although you might find an enlightened one that grills fish without batter.

Worst Choice:
➢ Everything aside from mushy peas

French Restaurants
Best Choice:
➢ Grilled meat
➢ Fish
➢ Vegetables
➢ Poultry

Worst Choice:
➢ Anything creamy or in a rich sauce or a cheese sauce
➢ Patés
➢ Anything in breadcrumbs

Burger Restaurants
Best Choice:
➢ Lean burgers
➢ Chicken burgers

Worst Choice:
➢ Chips
➢ Burger buns
➢ Fried full fat burgers

STOP! ACTION POINT!

Della's Eating Out Survival Guide
(eating out includes work canteens, tea shops, pubs…)

WORTH THREE STARS

Before you go out:
Make a copy of this page and take it with you.

When you're out:
- ➢ Choose clear vegetable or tomato based soups.
- ➢ Refuse bread.
- ➢ Ask for the butter to be left off vegetables/potatoes.
- ➢ Ask for sauces to be served separately.
- ➢ Choose tomato over cream based sauces.
- ➢ Choose stir fries.
- ➢ Choose chicken or fish, preferably grilled.
- ➢ Take your own fat free dressings.
- ➢ Make deals with yourself; wine _or_ dessert, starter _or_ dessert
- ➢ Ask for semi-skimmed milk with your coffee – or drink it black.
- ➢ Ask for chopsticks!

Changing The Way You Think

(Peter says…)

Never mind calorie counting, or spending your lunch hour on the treadmill, the real secret to eating loads and staying slim is to exercise the lump of grey matter between your ears, and to re-think your approach to food, *based on facts*.

And that's what this chapter is about. A few more thoughts about food and weight control that have the power to put you back in control of your waistline, all via a shift in mental gears.

So put those thinking caps on, and prepare to shed a few more pounds.

Acquiring Good Taste

(Della says…)

Food that tastes good tends to be bad for you – and food that isn't quite as appetising has an annoying habit of being slimmer friendly! Correct?

Well, not exactly!

It's perfectly possible to train yourself to not only *put up with* different tastes but to *prefer* them – which is extremely handy for an eat-loadser.

What we like, what tastes good to us and what tastes bad is one of those things that changes throughout our lives. It doesn't just change a little bit either. Surprisingly often, there can be a complete reversal.

Remember how you hated strong cheese as a child but grew to love it when you were in your thirties? Or maybe it's something else for you.

For me it was fish. I hated fish with a passion when I was small. It actually used to make me sick. I even had a note for school so I didn't have to eat it – I thought I was allergic to fish. So did my mother. Yet, today, I love fish. The change took place in my teens. I gave up meat when I was about sixteen. In those days it was incredibly hard to eat out if you didn't eat meat. So eventually, I started to eat fish. There was a fish option on most restaurant menus and I found, to my surprise, there were lots of types of fish I'd never tried that I really enjoyed.

I'd discovered by accident that it's possible to retrain your taste buds. Not just to change them a little but to actually completely reverse your likes and dislikes. These days, although I am no longer vegetarian, I eat fish three or four times a week.

Here's another example of retraining your taste buds that will probably ring bells with lots of people. For years I took sugar in hot drinks. I couldn't drink coffee or tea without it. Then I gave it up. I did this in one go – went cold turkey, so to speak, because personal experience has told me that going cold turkey, as opposed to cutting down gradually, is the most painless route to change for me. If you don't fancy this then you might prefer to try Peter's cutting down method mentioned in the More Swaps section earlier in the book.

For a short while I found it wasn't much fun having a hot drink without sugar. Then I grew used to it. Not long later I began to prefer it. Today, I couldn't drink a hot drink with sugar. It tastes awful. My tastes when it comes to sugar in hot drinks have completely reversed.

The same thing happened with milk. I switched from full fat to semi-skimmed. Then I switched to skimmed. Now I prefer my hot drinks with the smallest splash of skimmed milk. I'm not just putting up with the taste, I *prefer* it. I know countless people who have had this exact same experience. Maybe you're one of them. If you're not, try it. It's a completely pain-free way to cut calories.

STOP! ACTION POINT!

Re-train your taste buds

WORTH ONE STAR PER ITEM
(to a maximum of three stars)

Try one of the following:
 ➤ Give a food you 'don't like' another chance
 ➤ Reduce the amount of sugar, or milk, you usually have in hot drinks
 ➤ Swap a high fat food for a low fat alternative

Keep a Fully Stocked Fruit Bowl

(Della says…)

I mentioned fruit as a snack earlier – but it's not always the first thing you reach for, so this tip is a psychological slimming tip that has quite often worked for me.

Fill your fruit bowl with tangerines, apples, bananas and any other fruit you like, and then do a deal with yourself. The deal is this: You can go to the shop and buy a cream cake/chocolate bar/ice cream etc., but first you are going to eat three tangerines.

Very often by the time you have eaten the three tangerines you will find that your urge for something sweet has gone and you no longer want to race round to the shop for your cream cake. This really does work. And even if it doesn't, and you still want that cake, you might find you will make a better choice when you get to the shop. You will be in a better position to choose because your body won't be screaming *feed me sugar NOW, feed me sugar now!* You will also have eaten some of your five a day. Which has to be a bonus.

STOP! ACTION POINT!

Buy some fruit for your fruit bowl

ONE STAR FOR DOING THIS ONCE
ONE EXTRA STAR IF YOU DO IT REGULARLY
(..and eat the fruit!)

You don't have a fruit bowl? Well, it doesn't really matter; any glass bowl will do. Glass is good because you can see what you have. But a cooking dish will do at a push.

Now fill it with fruit. You don't even need to go out, although if you fancy some exercise then perhaps a walk to the shops could be good. But if you can only be bothered to walk as far as your computer, then why not order some fruit online? Here are two excellent organic suppliers who will deliver.

➢ http://www.abelandcole.co.uk/
➢ http://www.riverford.co.uk/

Waste or Waist?

(Peter says…)

Back in a previous chapter I made a passing reference to the fact that I was brought up to 'clear my plate'. There were, so I was told, starving children in Africa who would be only too happy to eat my mother's liver and bacon. And whilst my brother and I pointed out that we were happy to donate this particular meal to the starving children, it soon became apparent that not only was this not an option, but food we were refusing to eat would be served up every meal time, cold, until we'd eaten it.

Which is precisely what happened.

On more than one occasion.

Eventually we got the message:

**LEAVING FOOD IS A WASTE.
AND WASTE IS WRONG.**

And so began a lifetime of ensuring my plate was cleared. As kids we used to joke that my dad was 'the human dustbin' – able to eat his dinner and all our leftovers. But by the time I was married I too was routinely eating more than one large dinner every single evening: mine *and* whatever Kate had left.

You might be wondering (although I suspect many of you aren't) how I managed to do this. Why was there never a moment when I was just too full to finish my own food, let alone my wife's?

Part of the reason is undoubtedly because my internal fatometer (from earlier in the book, remember?) was probably very high, therefore maintaining a huge appetite, but there might have been another psychological process at work too. According to scientists, when it comes to 'eating loads' people use their eyes, not their stomachs, to determine how much that is.

In one such study (link on our website), scientists took fifty-four volunteers and sat them down to eat a bowl of soup. Whilst half of the participants ate from 'normal' soup bowls, the other half unknowingly ate from bowls that were rigged in such a way that they could be slowly re-filled without the diner realising it. These folks ate, on average, a staggering 73% more soup and, more interestingly, had no idea that they'd done so. The scientists concluded that when it comes to figuring out how much we've eaten we rely on what our eyes are telling us.

This is backed up by a famous experiment where cinema goers were able to eat significantly more popcorn than usual if they were given a bigger bucket – even if, astonishingly enough, the popcorn itself was several days old! Yuk!

This being the case, there are three relatively simple mental changes we can make which should have quite an impact on the amount of food that we eat.

Gut instincts – stop eating when you're full
Firstly, from here on, when it comes to food pay attention to your stomach. If you feel full, particularly if you're no longer enjoying the meal – stop eating! So there's still food on the plate. So what?

But what about those starving children in Africa? That's a very good point. Which is why you'll find a donation button to one of the numerous charitable organisations working in that part of the world on our website. Believe me, sending those organisations the odd donation will do you, and them, more good than forcing down food you don't need to eat.

Eat your food. No one else's
Secondly, do not finish other people's food. Ever. This is a really, really bad habit to get into. Whether you're finishing your wife's meals, or your kids', no good can come of it, and contrary to what your parents drilled into you, throwing away uneaten food is not a waste. Not in the grand scheme of things. How do I know this? Because I've checked.

Part of the reason I used to finish Kate's meals was because I'd started to obsess about how much food we threw away. As a single man I would quite often live on toast, or takeaways, simply because I couldn't be bothered to do a proper food shop – but once married, food shopping became a regular fortnightly event. The plus side of this new-found marital routine was that I no longer stared into an empty fridge and wondered if I could conjure a meal out of nothing; the downside was that my bin now seemed to be full of things that had gone out of date before we'd had a chance to eat them. Things that I had paid for. That was my money, sitting amongst the trash!

Most people would be content to let this gnaw away at their soul, occasionally allowing the frustration to ignite a row with their partner along the lines of "Why did you buy this if you had no intention of eating it?"Indeed I probably did both those things – but me being me, I also wanted to know exactly how much that rotting cabbage had cost me.

So, over a six week period, and using the itemised bill from our last online shopping delivery, I diligently highlighted all the items that Kate… and I… had thrown away. I then keyed the results into a spreadsheet, totalled up the wastage, and prepared to confront my wife.

The result astonished me.

In six weeks we'd thrown away a mere three pounds and thirty-six pence worth of food.

Three pounds.

And thirty-six pence.

Most of it vegetables.

Turns out the only waste you should be worrying about is the one spelt W.A.I.S.T.

The final tip we can take away from this section is that just as the scientists were able to make people eat more without them realising it, you too can reduce the amount you and your family eat without your brain registering the fact. How? By buying smaller plates.

Seriously.

Of course, I realise that this third idea will be instantly dismissed by most of you on the grounds that you can't afford to buy a replacement set of crockery. So let me put it to you this way. Right now I'm looking at a fifty piece porcelain dinner set, on amazon.co.uk, for £49.99. That's at the top end of the dinner sets available – most are significantly less. Does a one off payment of fifty pounds (max) really seem that expensive for something that will ultimately reduce what you eat by 10% without you even noticing it? How about a quick visit to your favourite online kitchenware store, before we move on?

One final word before you rush off and do that. Your replacement plates shouldn't be too much smaller than your existing plates. It still needs to look like a full size plate for your mind to accept it. Using a side-plate for your main meal won't actually work. So if you're using 10 inch plates, switch to 9.

Time for some action.

STOP! ACTION POINT!

Fool your eyes

WORTH TWO STARS

Seriously consider buying slightly smaller plates. They're not that expensive and over time you'll reduce the amount you eat by roughly ten per cent without even realising it.

Two new rules to live by:

WORTH ONE STAR EACH
(two in total)

1. When you're full, stop eating.
2. If it's not on your plate, don't eat it.

You don't have to clear your plate. Don't worry about the waste – worry about your waist.

Surviving Sabotage

(Della says…)

I remember once confiding to a close friend that I was planning to lose some weight. Her immediate reaction was to wrinkle up her nose and say, "So you're going to be boring and not eat any puddings."

"I suppose I am," was my reply, but I remember feeling a little taken aback. Was I going to be boring? I mean, who wants to be boring? What was the alternative – was it to listen to her and to eat a pudding I didn't actually want?

It's surprising how much of this kind of reaction you encounter when you decide to change things in your life (and not just your weight – but that's another story!) I'm not sure why it happens. A psychologist friend of mine says it's because humans don't like change. We don't like anything that threatens the status quo.

Maybe my friend thought I would expect her to stop eating puddings too. Maybe she would feel threatened if I lost weight and she didn't. Maybe she thought it would change how I felt about her. Maybe it was something she wanted to do herself but was too scared of trying in case she failed. It doesn't really matter what her reasons were but this is an attitude I've encountered a lot when I've tried to lose weight. Here are some of the comments I've heard from family, friends and, in some cases, from complete strangers.

> ➤ You don't need to lose weight, there's nothing of you.
> ➤ Wait till you get to my size before you bother with that.
> ➤ You're a pretty girl; don't waste time worrying about your weight. Enjoy life.
> ➤ You expect to put on weight once you hit forty, fifty, sixty etc.

Well, what if I don't want to wait until I'm any fatter? Maybe I think that a stone or two will be easier to shift than four stone. Maybe I think I will enjoy life more if I'm at the weight I'd like to be at. And maybe I don't accept that putting on weight as I age is an inevitable outcome.

If you want to lose weight, even if it's just a few pounds, then start now. And don't let anyone sabotage you.

"You're not fat darling, just have a tiny piece…"

Some would-be saboteurs aren't quite as subtle. If you have the type of family who will fill up the fridge with tempting treats as soon as you say you want to lose weight, or offer to get a takeaway, then you have my sympathies. Perhaps you could sit down with them and explain what you are trying to do and why.

Perhaps you can even get them on board. It's much easier to lose weight – or to stay at your ideal weight – if you're not trying to do it alone.

One of the best strategies, I've found, is also the most simple. Don't tell anyone you're trying to lose weight. Then they can't try and talk you out of it or do anything else to put you off.

STOP! ACTION POINT!

An anti sabotage strategy – don't mention the diet!

WORTH ONE STAR

Be firm. Don't say, "I can't have a dessert, I'm on a diet." This can be an open invitation to prospective saboteurs. Try saying, "I'm too full for a dessert."

No one is likely to argue with that one.

The Power of Focus

(Peter says…)

Brains are amazing. Especially yours. Even mine has its moments. And one of the most fascinating mechanisms of the human brain is how it deals with 'focus'.

Have you ever noticed how when you buy a new car, or even when you've merely decided what type of car it is you want to buy, you start seeing that same car everywhere?!

Or how you can sleep through a thunderstorm, the traffic noise, and the sounds of revellers returning from a night on the town, but if your newborn's breathing changes even slightly – *in the next room* – you're awake!

Or how you can see someone across a crowded room, start to walk towards them, and somehow collide with the table, the person, the immoveable object that was directly in front of you but momentarily invisible?

That's the power of focus. It happens because in order for our brains to cope with the extraordinary amount of information coming in through our five senses from the world around us, we're programmed to concentrate on what's 'important' and pretty much ignore the rest. So you probably won't be that surprised to learn that this mental focus mechanism can have a huge impact on the amount you eat and your ability to control your weight.

For instance, there have been a number of studies to show that people who are distracted whilst eating (i.e. focusing on something other than their food) tend to eat more. In one experiment (link on the website), people who listened to a detective story during their lunch break ate, on average, fifteen per cent more than usual.

So can we use this power of focus to help regain control over our weight? You betcha.

One of the most effective ways to control your weight and shed some pounds is merely to monitor what you eat, and when you eat it. The very act of noting down every item that passes your lips would constantly refocus your mind on how much you're eating, and your food choices in general.

Of course, being a man, a self-confessed nerd, and a list junkie, the real reason this idea appeals to me is because there's likely to be a phone app out there to facilitate this very task. And indeed there is! Several, in fact. Many of which are free, and have built-in functions to calculate the number of calories you're consuming. Hours of playing with your phone whilst engaging the awesome power of focus can be yours for the taking.

But before you run off to the app store, let's have a recap.

STOP! ACTION POINT!

Focus, dammit!

WORTH ONE STAR

When eating alone, focus on your food. No watching telly, no listening to the radio, no reading a magazine. Just eat.

WORTH THREE STARS

Get into the habit of keeping a food diary. Whether you jot items down in the back of your filofax, email yourself, or download an app doesn't matter, you'll still be bringing your focus back to your food, and food choices.

Food Advice

(Peter says...)

Earlier in the book Della told us that there have been studies that suggest chillies have the ability to increase the body's metabolism. Good news if you're a chilli fan, bad news if one drop of chilli sauce will have you rolling on the floor, red faced, eyes bulging in their sockets, whilst you gasp for someone to bring you some water.

But it's not just chillies that allegedly help the body burn fat. There are quite a few foods which purport to have similar magical properties, causing Della and me to debate whether we should include a list in this book.

Let's take a closer look at some of these so-called super foods.

Broccoli

One of my personal favourites when it comes to vegetables, broccoli is high in calcium and vitamin C, both of which are thought to help the body reduce excess weight.

Then again, broccoli – like most vegetables – contains virtually zero fat. If the broccoli on your plate replaces something less wholesome it's almost inevitable that you'd put on less weight – regardless of whether calcium or vitamin C are actually able to rid you of excess pounds.

One to add to your shopping list.

Water

Your average humble glass of water, consumed several times a day, has apparently been proven to boost your metabolism, promote weight loss, flush out toxins, reduce hunger, and make you more attractive to the opposite sex (I may have made one of those items up).

One thing is certain, however; it's a lot better for you than a can of coke.

Super fruits

Allegedly, one study found that participants who ate half a grapefruit with each meal lost, on average, three and a half pounds over a twelve week period. Another study in Rio de Janeiro found that dieting women who ate three small apples or pears a day lost more weight than those who followed the diet with no added fruit.

Was it down to the vitamin C again? Some other magical compound found only in apples or grapefruit? Or simply the fact the fruit replaced a chocolate bar?

Omega 3

According to some sources, omega 3 fatty acids are the mortal enemy of leptin. Leptin, as you may remember from the chapter How Hunger Really Works, is a hormone – and one of its many jobs is, apparently, to slow down your metabolism which, as any dieter will tell you, is bad news if you're trying to burn calories.

More omega 3, so the theory goes, less leptin. More metabolism, less weight.

Whether this is true or not isn't really relevant. There are far better reasons to top up your Omega 3 fatty acids than weight loss. For starters they're proven to make you smarter and less stressed, and those are good enough reasons for me.

You'll find omega 3 in abundance in oily fish such as mackerel (though not tinned tuna), fish oil tablets, or my personal favourite, hemp milk.

Garlic

It doesn't just prevent colds and blood clots whilst repelling vampires and other blood sucking midges, it also – so numerous articles on the internet will have you believe – breaks down fats!

Personally, the fact that it makes food taste absolutely wonderful, especially when combined with chilli and ginger, is reason enough for me to put it in every meal possible.

It's worth mentioning that I compiled this list in just a few minutes from various internet-based sources, many of which simply regurgitate information from other websites, often word for word. Few actually name the original source or the study on which the conclusions are drawn, which for me sets off alarm bells.

For instance, you could add *vinegar* to this list. Vinegar has been proven to reduce fat in laboratory mice and all the signs are that it should have the same effect in humans. However, mice are, by their very nature, quite small. So whilst the quantities of vinegar involved in the experiments might seem quite reasonable, to produce the same fat-burning results in humans you or I would have to drink pints of the stuff, which is clearly ridiculous! But in some articles it's common for essential information like this to be played down or dropped entirely, intentionally or otherwise.

My top tips on gathering weight-loss information from the internet would be as follows:

1) Beware descriptive words like 'massive', 'huge', 'incredible'. They make an article more interesting to read, but are not so great at communicating actual facts.

2) Look for the numbers. How many pounds were actually lost? Over what period? How many people were in the study? When did this take place? That 'grapefruit' study (where participants who ate half a grapefruit with each meal lost, on average, three and a half pounds over a twelve week period) really isn't that impressive when you think about it.

3) Seek out the source. Does the article mention the original scientific study? The name of the scientist involved? Maybe even the scientific journal in which the results were published? Without these details you could be reading nothing more than hearsay.

4) Finally, if something sounds too good to be true –
   especially if it fails points 1, 2 and 3 above – then
   I'm afraid it probably is.

Let's incorporate this into our mental arsenal.

STOP! ACTION POINT!

Food advice!

WORTH ONE STAR

When you hear new food advice, get into the habit of checking the following:
- ✓ Is there an overuse of emotionally charged, but unquantifiable, descriptive words?
- ✓ Does the advice come complete with numbers? (How much, how many, how long…)
- ✓ Is the advice based on a scientific study (that you can look up)?
- ✓ Does it sound too good to be true?

Myths About Weight Loss

(Della says...)

While we are on the subject of food advice, let's see if we can bust some myths about weight loss.

Way back in the days when we sat around a mammoth buffet with our old friends, Ug and Uggetta, being overweight wasn't an issue. The word diet hadn't even been invented back then. But you can bet your bottom dollar (or the currency of the day – maybe pebbles?) that the moment it came into existence, a whole host of diet myths sprung up around it, most of them started by people who were making assumptions based on half truths.

I'm sure you know most of these diet myths already. Several are bandied about every time a discussion about slimming begins – these are usually in the pub, I find! Some of them are patently ridiculous, for example: "You can only lose weight if you live on salad" – but some of them are less obvious. They sound like they might just be true, and they're the ones we're going to address in this section, as well as our own experiences, and fact-finding quests, all in an effort to separate myth from reality.

The time of day you eat makes a difference

I don't know where I got the idea that it was impossible to stay slim unless you ate your meals at certain times of day, but for years I was convinced this was the case.

I believed that one of the reasons I put on weight after I married was because my husband and I ate our main meal of the day so late. We worked long hours and if we wanted to eat together we would rarely make it to the table before nine p.m. More usually it was after ten.

The theory behind this myth sounds *almost* logical. The later you eat, the less time you have to work off the extra calories (because at bedtime they settle around your middle and become fat). This doesn't actually make any sense at all if you think about it. If you eat three meals totalling, for example, 1500 calories in a twelve hour period it doesn't matter whether you eat them earlier or later, or all three at once – you still have the same amount of time to burn them off. A surplus of calories is what creates fat.

The last (and hopefully final) time I lost two stone, I regularly ate my evening meal after ten p.m. I still do. And while it might not be the most ideal time from a digesting-your-food-properly point of view, it does not make the slightest bit of difference to your weight. I know several shift workers – nurses, firemen and factory workers – who can testify to this fact.

It is the total amount of calories you eat, not *when* you eat that makes the biggest difference to losing weight.

You must exercise to lose weight
You do not have to exercise in order to lose weight, although it can help. However, exercise on its own does

not make a significant enough difference to warrant the effort involved. You need to change the way you eat as well.

And I should know. I've conducted numerous exercise/weight loss experiments. Unlike Peter, I happen to like exercise; it has a lot of health benefits. It tones my muscles, it improves my skin, it makes me feel good (afterwards, not during) and it makes me feel virtuous (during and afterwards). But I have tried several times to lose weight by eating the same amount and upping my exercise levels significantly. It doesn't work.

When I was at my heaviest, thirteen stone seven (192 pounds), I decided to up my running from around eight miles a week to twenty-four miles a week (not all at once, I hasten to add) and over the course of a couple of months this made very little difference to my weight.

Here's another example. When I was thirty I ran in a race called The Dorset Doddle – obviously named by someone who has a great sense of humour. The distance is around thirty-one miles and the route is along the Dorset coast path, which goes up and down, and up and down, and up and down – it's probably only about three miles as the crow flies! A doddle it most certainly is not!

When I got home, and had recovered from the shock of so much exercise, I had a large takeaway curry to reward myself. Surely I had already burned off the calories. But no – it would seem not.

The next day I was a pound heavier! And yes, this did disappear again. But these experiences, and several others like them, have led me to believe that extreme exercise is not a very effective or swift way of losing weight. Once I have lost the weight exercise does help me to maintain it, and as I've mentioned, exercise has a lot of other benefits. So don't give up on it if you like it – but if you're like Peter and you don't then you can breathe a sigh of relief.

(Peter says...)

Talking of exercise, I saw a TV interview recently where a channel swimmer was explaining how he lost an entire stone in weight during the thirteen hours it took him to swim the twenty-something miles that separates us from France.

Initially I thought, "One stone – wow!" – but the more I thought about it the more I came to the conclusion that if it takes *thirteen hours* of continuous, gruelling exercise (without, one assumes, any kind of sustenance other than the occasional glucose drink administered from a guy in a boat) to lose perhaps ten per cent of your body weight, is it any wonder that my half hour jog, five days a week, failed to produce any noticeable results?!

Crikey! You can keep your Dorset Doddle.

Skip meals
(Della says...)

Actually, this one used to work quite well when I was younger. If I wanted a flat stomach for an evening out, skipping dinner the previous night was quite effective. It only really works if you're quite slim already though. It doesn't work at all as a long term weight-loss strategy.

One of the reasons it doesn't work is because you will probably feel deprived if you skip meals and are likely to play catch-up, by either eating more for your next meal or by grabbing a snack or two to compensate (especially if you're like me and can convince yourself that snacks aren't proper meals, and therefore don't count).

If you actually skipped meals regularly without catching up then this method of dieting would probably work fine. Any method of losing weight that means you're taking in less calories than you require should work fine.

However, personally I find I'm bad tempered when I'm hungry, which means it's not a method I would use. In actual fact, if I want to lose weight, I actually do the opposite to skipping meals; I have meals more often because this stops me feeling hungry. As I mentioned above, it's *what* you eat (in terms of calories) that's important. It doesn't matter when you eat them or over how many meals your calories are divided.

And, of course, this book is about staying slim and eating loads. So forget skipping meals – especially breakfast.

Avoid combining proteins and starches
(Peter says...)

Many, many years ago, back when I was in my teens, and long before fad diets had gathered enough popularity to be labelled 'fad' – I had a girlfriend (I know – it's hard to believe, but keep reading) who stumbled across a book about 'food combining' and its amazing ability to improve your digestion and help you shed pounds.

Pretty much from the moment she pulled that book from the shelf, every meal she ate came under intense scrutiny and was usually found 'wanting'.

'Food combining' is a complex subject and nowadays the term can be used to describe all kinds of eating disciplines that are designed to counter digestive or health problems. What they are, and whether they work, isn't up for debate – at least, not in this book. What does make me raise an eyebrow, however, is the idea that 'proteins and starches should never be eaten together'.

The argument goes something like this:

Proteins require an acidic environment to be digested, and starches the exact opposite (alkaline), so if your digestive system is faced with both, it has no idea what to do and the food just ends up sitting around, turning nasty and generally getting up to no good. This in turn leads to bloating, indigestion and weight gain.

Which all sounds very scary, and would be if it was based on anything resembling the truth.

Like a lot of food myths, the protein-starch-bad-combo myth is based on a misunderstanding of how the body works, and though the concept has become quite popular since it was first bandied around at the end of the 19th century, science has, in the meantime, gone on to discover *exactly* how your body digests foods. Not surprisingly, combining proteins and starches in the same meal, or even the same mouthful, isn't going to cause you the slightest problem.

Here's how your body works:

After you've swallowed your food it passes through the stomach, which soaks everything in acid to kill any harmful bacteria and begins breaking down the food for the next stage of digestion in the small intestine.

Here the stomach acid is neutralized, allowing an army of enzymes to deconstruct your food. There are different enzymes for fats, carbs, proteins – but regardless of what you eat, it's the same crack team of microscopic specialists that's responsible for deconstructing that meal and turning it into something the body can use.

In fact – and here's the kicker – most starches (such as rice, potatoes, bread, pasta), to a lesser or greater degree, contain a certain amount of protein. And foods that are high in protein (for example, beans and legumes) contain almost as many carbs. So any efforts to prevent proteins and starches sharing space on your dinner plate are pretty much doomed to failure.

Despite these facts my girlfriend did indeed lose weight when she was on her food combining regime, probably because if you're going to start dissecting every meal, picking and choosing what enters your mouth and what stays on the plate – particularly if those meals are prepared by someone else – it's almost inevitable that you'll end up eating less. But it certainly had nothing to do with how the body digests foods, that much we can prove.

Ready to earn more stars for making a minor mental gear change?

STOP! ACTION POINT!

Bust some myths!

WORTH ONE STAR

Challenge any pre-conceptions you have about food and weight loss. Try this. Write down everything you think you know about…

- ➢ Losing weight
- ➢ Fattening foods
- ➢ The way the body works

…then go check how true those assumptions actually are. You might be surprised.

How to Make Diets Work

(Della says…)

This is not a diet book, but I know that some of you may actually feel more comfortable with or prefer to try a more traditional diet. Ever started a diet and managed to do brilliantly well for the first day or two?

Chances are – if you're anything like me – you'll be so motivated that it almost seems easy at first. But by day three, or possibly towards the end of day two, your enthusiasm for being on a 'diet', especially if it has a lot of restrictions, may start to wane a little.

So this section is for you.

I've Had One So I've Blown It

(Della says…)

So, day seven of this damn diet, and it suddenly hits you that it'll be absolutely ages before you'll have lost any weight, which means that this denial thing is going to go on for a while. Too long.

Perhaps it wouldn't hurt to have just one biscuit, you tell yourself. That's a perfectly rational thought, isn't it? And you're right – it probably wouldn't hurt to have just one biscuit. So here's what you do. You reach for the packet, which may or may not be open. You get out just one biscuit. You put the other biscuits away again in the cupboard – up really high so they are less accessible. You put your single biscuit on a plate and you make a nice cuppa to go with it and then you nibble it slowly and really savour it.

Well, this is the theory, anyway. And maybe you are the sort of person who can do just that. But if you were you wouldn't have picked up this book. Perhaps your reality is more like mine – and it goes something like this. You grab the biscuits, eat one while you're waiting for the kettle to boil – who needs plates! Then you tip out another couple – they are quite small, and you hardly tasted that one anyway because you ate it so quickly.

Yes, you were going to have just one, but before you know it you've eaten four – well, you've blown it now, so you may as well finish the packet.

And as you've 'blown it', there suddenly doesn't seem to be any point in continuing with the diet at all. You may as well just give up and have a good blow out for the rest of the day too.

Perhaps, surprisingly, this is actually the point at where the diet was really blown. Because if you did decide to stay on the eating plan, whatever it was, then a packet of biscuits isn't the end of the world. It's not brilliant but it's not too much of a tragedy. If you were to actually go back to sensible eating afterwards, chances are you would probably still succeed.

So one of my tips to make traditional diets work is this: don't get into the 'I've blown it anyway so I may as well give up' mentality. Just put it down to experience and start again from that point on. Don't forget basic principle number six, as mentioned at the start of this book: healthy eating most of the time is usually good enough. Carry on with your planned meals. And don't beat yourself up because you're a human.

STOP! ACTION POINT!

You've not blown it till you've blown it!

WORTH ONE STAR
for mastering this concept

If you have a little wobble in your diet, simply continue with your smart eating strategy immediately afterwards.

Eat More If You're Dieting

(Della says…)

Grazing is a good habit to get into if you are trying to lose weight. I am defining grazing as eating little and often, as opposed to having two or three big meals a day.

Every time you eat a meal there is a slight raise in your metabolic rate[12], brought on by the actual process of eating and digesting your food – which means that for a while after eating, your body will burn calories at a faster rate. This is a very handy thing to know if you would like to burn calories faster with no other effort involved than eating more often. But remember to make smart choices.

Also, of course, eating little and often means you won't be so hungry, which means you're more likely to stick to a healthy eating plan and not to grab the first snack that takes your fancy. Not that it would matter if this was a fat free snack, of course!

Perhaps now would be a good time to refer to the list of savoury standby snacks you made earlier.

You did make a list, didn't you?

You will, of course, also have a bowl of fruit to hand, which you prepared earlier. Although I have found to my cost that if I happen to have a bowl of fruit handy and also a packet of crisps handy, I'll tend to veer towards the crisps because, well, let's face it, they are

---

[12] See our website for some interesting links to metabolic studies

much nicer and I want them more. Which brings me on to another of my top slimming tips – but first, action!

STOP! ACTION POINT!

Consider grazing

TWO STARS IF YOU DO IT REGULARLY

Try splitting your three main meals into four or five smaller meals. The important thing is not to increase the overall calories for that day.

Save The Best Till Last

(Della says…)

I find the worst thing about any kind of eating plan, particularly one that I'm going to incorporate into my life on a permanent basis, is the thought that I can't have 'something nice'.

'Something nice' – a treat – is different for everyone. For me, it tends to be something sweet. I have a very sweet tooth. An eating plan which doesn't allow sweet treats wouldn't work for me. I look forward to them. I enjoy looking forward to them. The downside of this is that once I've had them I've got nothing left to look forward to, so I tend to save them until later in the day.

There is nothing quite as satisfying as getting to teatime and thinking, ha ha, I still have something I really fancy for after tea. This isn't as important when you're just maintaining your weight – after all, you can have more than one treat anyway, then – but it's one of my top tips for losing weight successfully. It will be much easier to stick to your chosen slimming plan if you save the best till last.

For the purposes of this section I'm defining treat as something you can only have a limited amount of times. There are lots of fat free desserts you can eat as much of as you like – and interestingly, just because of this, you'll probably find you don't want to eat them to excess.

Your treat should be something you *can't* eat in unlimited quantities. I don't count calories, mainly because I'm not very good at adding up. Except when it comes to treats. This is because I can't think of a better system. Let me explain. One of my favourite treats is chopped banana, topped with a fat free thick yoghurt, which has a teaspoon of chocolate flavoured spread mixed through it. This has about 250 calories in it so it can, therefore, be swapped with something else that has 250 calories in it.

If cheese is your thing, then have a piece of cheese that is the same calorific value. By law the manufacturers of pre-packaged foods in the UK and other member states of the European Union must label the nutritional energy of their products in both kilocalories ('kcal') and kilojoules ('kJ'). Usually, the energy content of food is given for 100g and for a typical serving size. In countries and in situations where foods are not pre-packaged, weigh the food and check the calorific value in a book or website that exists for this purpose. It is also possible to buy kitchen scales that have types of food pre-programmed in, for example apples, and will give you the calories of the item.

If you prefer sweet things you might want to substitute a chocolate bar – cereal bars are good treat value. Often you can have two of them (particularly the light or low fat versions) for the same calorific value as a chocolate bar, for example. And again, the packets will be labelled so you don't have to work anything out.

I think it's quite important to have a treat every single day if you're actively losing weight. Alternatively, if you've got a special meal out or a social occasion you might want to save your treat allowance for that.

In order for the 'save the best till last' trick to stay effective, you will probably need to do one more thing. Like anything in life the novelty of a treat wears off when you have it too often. So vary the treat. Make sure it's something you really like, but the minute the shine starts to wear off, change it. It's quite good fun researching this.

STOP! ACTION POINT!

Save a treat till bedtime!

WORTH ONE STAR

Try saving your favourite treat till bedtime. If you're the type of person who can't stop at one then make sure your treat is a single item – not, for example, a chocolate biscuit from a pack of twenty.

Ring The Changes

(Della says…)

Another of the pitfalls of traditional diets can be that it's easy to get into the habit of continually eating the same kind of foods, particularly foods that are considered to be 'very healthy'. This can lead to you getting extremely bored and being tempted to give up on 'very healthy' foods. Not many people are content with eating the same things day in, day out, although I did once read about a man who ate cheese and pickle sandwiches on brown bread every single lunchtime for forty-five years. If this is you then great, it will certainly simplify things.

However, you might find it is more fun to ring the changes, particularly when choosing your main meals. Add a new meal to your repertoire regularly and you are unlikely to get bored.

I'm not suggesting you shouldn't ever repeat meals; once you've found meals you really love then it's handy to have them on a regular basis. But don't forget to plan new meals too.

One of the reasons so many restrictive diets fail is that as soon as the 'dieting' period is over, the slimmer drifts back to the eating patterns they had before, and these tend to be the eating patterns that made them put on weight. That's why dieting isn't usually a long term solution.

There is an added bonus for eat-loadsers too. Ringing the changes will help to lower your fatometer. So it's good news all the way.

STOP! ACTION POINT!

Plan a completely new meal

WORTH ONE STAR

You don't have a clue what to cook? You don't feel inspired to create something? Then do one of these things: invest in a low fat cook book; buy one of the slimming magazines that has recipes; or check out our website for our latest suggestions.

Do one of these things right now. Then add the ingredients to your weekly shopping list.

It doesn't have to be an evening meal. It could be a lunch or simply a new fat free snack!

The Cream Cake Conundrum

(Della says…)

Cream cake or apple? Which should you choose? Well, I guess the answer to this may depend on the following: are you watching your weight or aren't you? If you're not watching your weight then you can have the cream cake and if you are then I'm afraid it's the apple. Correct? Well, no actually – at least, not necessarily. I believe that – even if you are watching your weight – there can be a strong argument for choosing the cream cake. And yes, I know this completely contradicts what I said in the Keep A Fully Stocked Fruit Bowl section.

Why do I think you should sometimes choose the cake? Well, let's just consider the following scenario. This is day nine of the diet and you did brilliantly well yesterday. You've been doing brilliantly well for a while. You've been losing weight – you've started to see results – fantastic. You've also, slightly less fantastically, started to dream about cream cakes. In fact, you had one such dream last night, and now you can't get cream cakes out of your head.

Then you go to work and it's someone's birthday. It's always someone's birthday – and what happens on birthdays? Yes, cream cakes. Birthday Girl brings them in and flashes them around the office. For ages you've got around this by being armed with a healthy treat. This way when everyone else gets going on the cream cakes you don't feel quite as deprived because you've got your healthy treat.

Today you are armed with an apple. You don't want the apple – you want the cream cake. But you've been doing so well! You can't blow it now.

"Fancy a cream cake?" says Birthday Girl, flashing them under your nose. "There's a cream horn or a vanilla slice going begging."

Cream horns are your favourite.

"No, thanks." You grit your teeth, refuse the cream cake, refuse to even look in the pink cake box, refuse to breathe temporarily while the box passes by, so you can't even smell the cream cake.

Then you cut the apple into slices to make it last longer and then resolutely eat it.

Success. You have won another battle with temptation. You are amazing. In your previous life you were possibly even a saint! You give yourself a mental pat on the back. Pity you still can't get cream cakes out of your head but that's OK. You didn't eat one – you actually ate an apple.

The morning passes slowly. It is half an hour before lunchtime.

"Are you sure you don't fancy a cream cake?"

"What?" Your head jerks up. Hasn't that particular temptation passed? Hasn't that battle been won? Surely someone else hasn't brought in cream cakes.

No, it's the same pink box.

"There's just one left," Birthday Girl simpers. "Go on, treat yourself."

You feel yourself weakening. Please don't let it be the cream horn. The vanilla slice is refusable, but if it's the cream horn…

Birthday girl wafts the box under your nose. You close your eyes. It doesn't help. The delicious smell of cream cakes is calling to you. You open your eyes. It is of course the cream horn.

All thoughts of saying no leave your head. You grab the cake and shovel it into your mouth before you can change your mind. You swallow rapidly. You barely taste it. After it's gone you sit there feeling awful. You are not a saint, after all. You gave in. You are a bad person. You will now fail your diet. You will have put on at least three pounds before next weigh in.

None of this, of course, is true. What you have actually done is eaten more calories than you planned to do and you haven't enjoyed them.

Maybe, on this particular occasion, it would have been better to have chosen the cream cake in the first place. This is for three reasons.

- ➤ Chances are you wouldn't have eaten the apple as well so you'd have actually eaten fewer calories overall.
- ➤ You'd have enjoyed the cream cake, rather than guiltily shovelling it down.

➢ You wouldn't now be beating yourself up for being a miserable failure.

This is one of those occasions when it's probably better to look at the big picture. There are times when it's better to lose an individual battle if it means you're going to win the war. Which brings me on nicely to the last part of this section.

The Day Off Diet

(Della says…)

A friend of mine once told me that she and another friend attended a well known slimming club, which involved a weekly Thursday afternoon weigh in. They didn't take too much notice of the diet; each week they simply cut down on food radically on Mondays, Tuesdays and Wednesdays, in preparation for their weigh in. Which worked quite well for them as far as losing weight went (although probably isn't advisable as a long term strategy). Then on the way home, once the weigh in was safely out of the way, they bought fish and chips.

Now, I'm not advocating starvation as a good strategy. Nor buying fish and chips, come to that. But I do think it's a good idea to have a day off your diet. This is another one of those instances where winning the war is more important than winning an individual battle. It's really a numbers game, isn't it? Ultimately, if you take one day a week off your diet – you can eat whatever you like on this day – you will probably be able to stick to it for a lot longer, which overall will result in you losing more weight.

I should just finish this section, and indeed chapter, by saying that I'm not an advocate of diets at all. I think that changing the way you eat permanently is less stressful and ultimately more successful. But occasionally giving yourself completely free rein can be a very good thing.

The Strangest Diet Ever…

(Peter says…)

Remember how way back at the start of this book I told you how hunger really works? That you have an internal fatometer that determines a weight your body wants to be – and that you'll feel more hungry, more often, if your real weight is less than the fatometer – and less hungry, less often, if it's above? I went on to explain how your body associates calories with flavours, and will turn the fatometer up each time you eat anything with a strong calorie-flavour association.

This is pretty mind-boggling because if we follow this logically it means that if you consume calories, but no flavour – no flavour at all – your body should turn your fatometer *down*.

Which means that you'll feel less hungry, less often.
Which should mean that you'll eat less.
Which means you'll lose weight.
Which means you've just lost weight by eating!
Sounds crazy, doesn't it?
But it's entirely possible.

The Oil Diet

Welcome to possibly the strangest 'diet' in the western world. I've tried a few odd things over the years on my quest for 'eat loads and stay slim' nirvana, but this is probably the weirdest.

The first thing to understand is that the 'Oil Diet' isn't really a diet at all. It doesn't ask you to count calories. It doesn't ask you to limit the amount you eat. It doesn't forbid certain foods or food groups. It merely asks you to be really strict with yourself for two hours each day.

And to drink two tablespoons of a near-flavourless oil.

Della and I debated long and hard on whether this diet should be in the book. It definitely works because I've tried it, but how could we claim this book is diet-free if we've gone and included one – regardless of whether it's technically a diet in the truest sense of the word.

In the end we've compromised. It's here to illustrate how your fatometer works, but you get no stars for trying it. Think of this as a bonus section.

So here's what to do:

1) *Decide in advance what time each day you're going to do the diet.* You need two hours when you can be completely strict with yourself. What you eat or drink the rest of the day is completely up to you, but for those two hours make sure you follow these eight steps precisely. Most proponents of the diet tend to do it either first thing in the morning or last thing at night – that way you're asleep for one of those hours.

2) *Use a clock* – The first and final hour of this regime are there to prevent the calories in the oil from being associated with anything you might have eaten, or might eat, before or after. If you're used to snacking or drinking pretty much constantly throughout the day, these two hours can really drag (another reason why I like to be asleep for one of them). For this reason don't estimate the time – use a clock! You might find setting a reminder on your phone useful.

3) *Begin the first hour* – Stop eating and drinking. <u>Absolutely</u> <u>nothing</u> (with the exception of unflavoured water) can pass your lips. This hour is a buffer so that the calories in the next stage don't get associated with anything you may have eaten earlier. For the same reason you mustn't smoke, brush your teeth, chew gum, or do anything else that might involve a flavour. If you break this rule you risk triggering a flavour-calorie association which will raise your set-point, ultimately causing you to <u>GAIN</u> weight.

4) *Drink two tablespoons of a near flavourless oil* – Measure out a tablespoon (or two) of near-flavourless oil into a glass. Top up your glass with three or four times as much water, and then swallow the whole lot down immediately (don't leave the liquids to separate). It's nowhere near as unpleasant as you'd think. It should feel exactly like drinking a glass of water.

5) *The second hour* – Continue to abstain from all food, drink and anything other than plain unflavoured water, for another hour. Again, this is a buffer. Again use a clock.

6) *Be really, really strict with yourself* – I really can't stress this enough. This is probably the only diet which will ultimately make you gain weight if you screw it up!

7) *Do something else!* – You don't have to sit there on your hands with tape over your mouth. You can still read, watch TV, go for a walk, call a friend, go to the gym, listen to music, sleep!!

8) Repeat daily until you reach your target weight.

And that's it!

Which oil to use

Which oil you use is crucial to the success of the diet. Put away that extra virgin olive oil – that won't work. Neither will that fat free sunflower nonsense. The oil needs calories, but no flavour.

I use the 'mild & light' version of a popular brand of olive oil. It's mild and light in *flavour* – but the calories are the same as regular olive oil, which is very, very important. Apparently you can also try refined walnut oil, or refined coconut oil (the refining process reduces some of the flavour), light hemp oil, or safflower oil but I haven't done this myself as yet.

How and why the diet works

By following the steps above you're effectively introducing a large amount of 'flavourless' calories into the body. This prompts your body to turn your fatometer down.

As the days pass your fatometer will eventually fall below your real weight, making you feel less hungry, less often. Food cravings will vanish. Moderately sized meals will satisfy you completely. And as a result... you'll start to lose weight. Enough to counter the calories within the oil, and then some.

I'm not going to lie to you. I'm aware how completely bonkers this sounds.

When I first read about this 'diet' I was certain that it must be a ruse. Despite my cynicism I summoned the courage to give it a go.

For those first three weeks I didn't dare look at my bathroom scales for fear of seeing my weight creeping ever upwards. Eventually – utterly convinced that the person in the mirror hadn't lost a single ounce – I stood on the scales and prepared myself for an unpleasant shock.

I'd lost two pounds.

This made my head spin. Two pounds probably sounds like a pathetic amount of weight loss, and indeed it is, but I'd achieved it by doing, well – nothing! Yet despite consuming a vast number of calories every evening before switching off my bedside light, I'd somehow *lost weight.*

I continued and, to my considerable surprise, lost more weight. About a pound a week. For the first time ever I was starting to get slimmer.

The 'diet' actually worked.

Ever the sceptic, Della recently challenged me to repeat the oil diet.

I started on the 11th December 2012 when I weighed 13 stone 6lb. I took two tablespoons of 'mild & light' olive oil most evenings (skipping the week between Christmas and New Year, any evening when I went out for dinner (perhaps once a week) and a couple of weekends when I was away from home). Aside from the oil I ate 'normally'[13]. On the 10th February 2013 I was 13 stone exactly. A loss of six pounds over nine weeks, or one pound every ten days.

Possible side effects

The oil diet actually has a number of side effects. Here's a list of them, and what to do if you notice them.

> ➢ *Indigestion* – This hasn't happened to me but some people find that they suffer indigestion after drinking the oil. If this happens the advice

---

[13] I go into more detail about what's 'normal' for me at the end of the next chapter.

is to cut down on the quantity for a day or two. This gives your body time to develop the enzymes it needs to digest the oil.

➤ *Better skin* – Oddly, many people report better skin, less acne, silkier hair. If this happens be sure to toss your head to draw maximum attention to it, and to wear a smug expression at all times.

➤ *Better sleep* – Some people report better sleep (possibly because of the high omega 3 content in some oils). That's almost reason enough to give it a go.

➤ *Bloated feeling after eating* – A few days into the diet you might find that you feel bloated after eating – like you're going to explode[14]. This is actually the diet at work! Having lowered your set-point you'll feel fuller, faster. Meals that you once considered normal size are now too big. There are three solutions. Firstly, cut back the amount of oil you're using to one tablespoon for a day or two. Secondly, stop eating when you feel full. Finally serve less in the first place.

Frequently asked questions

➤ *Is the amount of oil important?* The amount of oil (and therefore calories) alters how quickly

---

[14] I've noticed this nearly always happens to me after pizza. I now skip the oil diet on pizza nights.

your fatometer falls below your real weight. For instance, reduce the amount of oil and your body will turn down your fatometer more slowly, but it also might not be enough to offset your fatometer-raising activities. On the other hand use more oil (three or four tablespoons) and I've found that you're more likely to feel bloated and ill after meals. For me, one or two tablespoons seems just right.

➢ *But a whole tablespoon!? That's a lot of calories!!* Yes. It is. However, do the diet right and the rest of the day you'll consume fewer calories than you gain from the oil. Think of it as 'one step back, two steps forward' on the road to achieving your target weight.

➢ *How fast will I lose weight?* Slowly. About a pound a week, which is generally considered a healthy rate of weight loss.

➢ *Is there anything I can do to make it work faster?* Actually, yes. Here are a few ideas:

✓ Eat normally. Don't use the diet as an excuse to eat like a pig at every meal (the old 'I went to the gym at lunchtime therefore I can have this chocolate bar and all the others in the vending machine' gambit). The diet's really good at reducing your appetite, and in my experience even better at making you feel full. If you work against it by stuffing your face more than usual you'll only feel ill. (This is the voice of experience talking!)

✓ Eat when you're hungry. If you want to eat, eat. If you don't, don't! Trust your body.

✓ Employ the other techniques in this book. Without hunger bothering you every five seconds you'll probably find the other techniques in this book easier to adopt, and therefore doubly as effective.

Monitor your progress

I'm not a big fan of daily weighing – in my experience that kind of weight monitoring causes you to obsess about your weight and food, which in turn focuses your mind on the wrong thing. However, because of the way the diet works, and because – if you get it wrong – it can cause you to gain weight rather than lose it, it's probably a good idea to weigh yourself approximately once a week, at the same time[15]. If you notice (after a couple of weeks) that you're gaining weight, stop the diet. Before giving the diet another go, have another read of the eight step process and check that you're following it to the letter.

---

[15] An excellent phone app for monitoring and charting your weight – thereby accounting for any 'blips' – is True Weight. Other apps are available.

Find out more

I thoroughly recommend Doctor Seth Roberts' book (The Shangri-La Diet[16]) which covers all of the above and much, much more.

---

[16] ISBN-13: 978-0340922569.

Putting It All Together

(Peter says...)

So how are you? How are you feeling? Slender? No? Why not? What have you been doing for the last goodness knows how many pages – sitting on your backside, reading? Don't tell me you've been ignoring the Action Points! Tch! What are you like!

Well fear not. As the saying goes, "the show ain't over till the fat lady sings," and this chapter is intended to make sure that there is no fat lady. Or gentleman. Grab a pen and a piece of paper (for real this time) and prepare to start making lots of small changes to your life.

Peter & Della's Top Tips for Losing Weight

(Peter & Della say...)

Right then troops, listen up. Pens at the ready? Good. What follows are our top-tips for eating loads, but staying slim, boiled down to a few easy steps.

Aim never to be hungry

Hunger is the enemy.

- ➤ Reduce your appetite by avoiding foods that turn up your fatometer, and keep your fatometer down low by mixing up flavours and trying new foods as often as possible (see the chapter '*How Hunger Really Works*').
- ➤ Try using the oil water diet to lower your fatometer. Make sure you follow the guidelines precisely.
- ➤ Grazing on low fat or fat free food is good on many levels. It will stop you ever getting hungry enough to blow your healthy eating regime and it will give you a helpful metabolic boost.

Choose food carefully

Ask yourself a question: is it worth the calories? If it isn't, don't eat it. See 'Smart Food Choices'.

Also, you really don't need to eat meat every meal. Vegetables are actually amazing! Just mix 'em up to make them interesting. See '*This Chapter is Not About Vegetables*'.

Swaps

Use swaps to painlessly change your less healthy food habits.

Try swapping high fat for low fat or fat free, especially when cooking. (OK, this is Della's top tip, not Peter's.) And if you can find a low fat or fat free food that tastes as good as a high fat food, it won't even be painful to swap. What's not to like?

Plan what you eat

Forward thinking and planning is the ultimate secret to gaining control over your weight. (See '*Planning*' in the chapter '*Smart Food Choices*'.)

Know your snacking danger zones

Keep some fat free snacks available at all times. Make sure they are snacks you really, really fancy. Make sure they do not require any more effort than popping in your mouth. Snacks you have to actually cook (unless you cook them in advance) are a no no.

Compromise on calories, but not on taste

The reason you're drawn to 'bad' food is because it just tastes better! So let's 'level the playing field' and improve the flavour of the foods we should be eating.

Herbs, chillies, spices, garlic all make food taste good. Mix them up and tantalise your taste buds.

When you are full, stop eating
Trust your gut. Are you eating merely because it's there? When you're full, stop eating – and throw the rest away. And next time serve a smaller portion. On smaller plates. (See the chapter '*Changing The Way You Think*'.)

If it's not on your plate, don't eat it
Finishing everyone else's meals will not, sadly, make one jot of difference to world poverty. It might seem like a waste, but in the grand scheme of things it really isn't. What it is, is extra W.A.I.S.T. (See the chapter '*Changing The Way You Think*'.)

Della's low fat cooking principles!
   ➢ Use a low fat cooking spray for frying and roasting
   ➢ Only use extra lean meat
   ➢ Trim visible fat from meat
   ➢ Swap sugar for sweetener
   ➢ Swap cream for fat free fromage frais or yoghurt
   ➢ Where milk is mentioned in recipes use semi-skimmed or skimmed
   ➢ Always have fat free treats in the fridge to snack on while cooking
   ➢ Where cheese is mentioned, use half fat
   ➢ Ban butter

➢ Keep a fat free salad dressing made up in the fridge

Totalling Your Star Rating

(Peter & Della say...)

So back to those golden stars. How did you do? If you haven't been totting them up as you've gone along, grab a pencil and let's do that now.

Buying this book
     - worth 1 star

Basic Principles
Commit to making changes
     - worth 1 star

How Hunger Really Works
Understand the fatometer
     - worth 1 star
Keep your fatometer as low as possible
     - worth 1 star

Smart Food Choices
Smart breakfasts
     - worth 1 star per breakfast, to a maximum of 2
Smart snacking!
     - worth 1 star per snack, to a maximum of 3
Food swaps
     - worth 1 star per swap, to a maximum of 5
Plan three meals
     - worth 2 stars per meal, to a maximum of 6

Vegetables
Give vegetables a chance – try it out
   - worth 1 star
Turn semi veggie
   - worth 7 stars
Herbs and hot stuff – try it out
   - worth 1 star
Herbs and hot stuff – stick to it
   - worth 1 star

Surviving Social Eating
Master the eating out survival guide
   - worth 3 stars
Retrain your taste buds
   - worth 1 star
Buy some fruit for your fruit bowl – once
   - worth 1 star
Buy some fruit for your fruit bowl – regularly
   – worth 1 star

Changing the Way You Think
Switch to smaller plates
   - worth 2 stars
When you're full, stop eating
   - worth 1 star
If it's not on your plate don't eat it
   - worth 1 star
Don't mention the diet – Della's anti sabotage strategy

- worth 1 star
Focus on your food
- worth 1 star
Keep a food diary
- worth 3 stars
Vet food advice
- worth 1 star
Bust some myths
- worth 1 star

How To Make Diets Work
You've not blown it till you've blown it
- worth 1 star
Consider grazing
- worth 2 stars
Save a treat till bedtime
- worth 1 star
Plan a completely new meal
- worth 1 star

There are a total of fifty four stars on the table! The more you've earned, the higher your chances of being able to eat loads and stay slim.

Interestingly, you don't actually need to score that high in order to notice a difference. In a page or two's time we'll reveal our star ratings, but in the meantime here's a rough and ready guide.

0-14 stars

We're going to assume you must be ultra slender already and with a constitution that allows you to eat a tub of lard without consequences, and that's why you've decided to read this far without actually doing anything.

15-28 stars

Hmmm. You're doing, er OK, ish, but you probably need to earn a few more stars if you want to see long term results.

29-41 stars

Well done you. You should already be seeing some really good results, and be well on the way to permanently eating loads and staying slim.

42-54 stars

Wow! You little (slim) star you! Fancy being on the cover of the second edition?

Peter's
How To Eat Loads and Stay Slim
Star Rating is:
32

Della's
How To Eat Loads and Stay Slim
Star Rating is:
44

How Peter Eats Loads and Stays Slim

(Peter says)

It's been a while since I stood on my bathroom scales.

Actually, that's not quite true. I needed to weigh myself earlier in the book so I could tell you how heavy I am, and in order to do that I first had to find the bathroom scales, and then find a battery to replace the one that had long since died. Weight isn't something that bothers me any more. I'm back to how life was in my twenties. Eating what I want, when I want, and not really thinking about the consequences.

Almost.

The truth is I've retrained myself. Made many, many changes to the way I eat so that what I *want* to eat is no longer going to accumulate in places that I don't want it to. Here's a summary of my eating habits.

For starters I'm *almost* a vegetarian. Unless I'm cooking for friends, or eating out, most meals I prepare are meat-free. Every three or so weeks I have a box of organic fresh vegetables delivered and I aim to use everything, even if I have to take a picture and post it on Facebook to find out what on earth some of the vegetables actually are.

I eat out about once a week, and probably cook for someone once a week too. At these times I stick rigidly to Basic Principle number 6:

HEALTHY EATING,
MOST OF THE TIME,
IS USUALLY GOOD ENOUGH

In other words I pig out on whatever I want when I'm out because the rest of the week is 'most of the time' (remember: as an author I work from home). That said, I'm a real 'foodie', and enjoy the opportunity of eating out to try something new, which you'll remember is very important.

Back home again I don't use fat free anything. It's actually one of the few things Della and I really don't agree on. Semi-skimmed milk is the closest I ever get.

I adore cheese, and bread, but I try ('try' being the word) not to rely on these favourites too much. To make bread nutritionally better (though sadly, not less fattening) I use a bread maker, wholemeal flour and invent my own bread recipes[17]. Thinking about it, this probably changes the flavour of the bread, thereby keeping my fatometer low, but I could be stretching the point somewhat.

Nutrition is quite a big deal for me. Swap your obsession with 'fat free' foods, for 'nutrient rich'. Treat

---

[17] Here's one: 1.25 teaspoons of yeast. 550g of strong wholemeal flour. 2 teaspoons of sugar. One 25g knob of butter. 1.5 teaspoons of salt. Two eggs topped up to 390ml with hemp milk. 1 handful of chopped sun dried toms. One quarter of a large onion. One chopped green chilli or a sprinkle of dried chilli flakes. Into the bread maker. Press GO.

it like a game: how nutritionally significant can I make this meal?

I bulk cook! Unless I'm entertaining I never want to spend longer cooking than I do eating. The only way to do this is to cook big dishes (I mean huge – literally as large as I can) that can be divided into portions and frozen. It's great knowing that there's a freezer full of fat free meals. Now that's planning!

I usually have a glass of wine each evening. Pizza is still my favourite meal (home-made, including the base). And I still eat burgers but they're veggie burgers, and more often than not home-made by my friend Wendy, who's a truly wonderful cook. Not sure she'll make any for you though.

And finally, if I stand in front of the mirror naked and I'm not happy with how I look I set a daily alarm on my phone and start doing the Oil Diet every night until I'm happy again.

How Della Eats Loads and Stays Slim

(Della Says)

Well, I do get on my bathroom scales fairly regularly. Usually to check if my favourite jeans have actually shrunk in the wash – there's always the faint hope – or whether I've been a little too lax in sticking to my 'eat loads and stay slim' principles. OK, then, you've caught me out – I mean ignoring them altogether.

In the unlikely event that the jeans have shrunk I carry on blithely as I am.

In the much more likely event that I have actually put on a few pounds then I have a quick reassessment of how things have been lately. Have I been eating out too much and not making smart choices, but tucking into the home-made bread and butter pudding my favourite pub makes too often? Have I been grabbing snacks (like chocolate) that cannot be classified as fat free on a more regular basis than usual? Have I perhaps been ignoring my fat free cooking principles?

It's usually one of the first two; the third one is pretty much second nature and it's also the easiest one to stick to.

Next I have a quick think – am I happy with the way things are? Shall I buy bigger jeans? Usually the answer to these two questions is no. Why don't I just wear my stretchy leggings with the elasticated waistband instead?!

But I jest. While I may wear my stretchy leggings for a week or so, my primary objective now becomes to get back into my favourite jeans. I love being slim. I love eating loads. I know it is possible, with a little thought and planning, to do both.

I usually kick-start my regime again by doing two things: the first is to cook a fat free meal I really, really like. Chances are I won't have had it lately or I wouldn't have put on any weight, so it'll be a novelty again. The second thing I do is to find or invent a brand new fat free meal that I fancy trying. Quite often, this will be a conversion of something I've had and really enjoyed somewhere, but using my fat free cooking principles – the ones we've discussed in this book.

Usually it does not take very long to get back into my jeans and it's relatively painless. Losing a few pounds when I need to is far easier than losing a few stone. And it's so worth it. I promise.

And – here's a point to ponder – writing this book has made me aware that I have all the tools I need to succeed. You're reading it – so you have them too.

You Still Here?

Peter's Final Remarks

These past few years have been some of the best and happiest in my entire life. I reached forty and had another growth spurt – a mental one, rather than physical – and of all the things I've learnt there appears to be a common theme: there is no 'normal'.

To put that into the context of this book, you might believe, as I did, that it's 'normal' to put on weight. Particularly as you get older. That it's 'normal' to be in a constant state of weighing up what you *want* to eat with what you *should* eat. Maybe you've even got to the point where you believe it's 'normal' to be overweight, 'normal' not to be happy with how you look, 'normal' that the you in your head and the you in the mirror are two entirely different people.

It's not normal.

Or at least, it doesn't have to be *your* normal.

You can change everything.

Not overnight, and not without some effort, but you can change *everything*.

Smarter food choices, eliminating hunger, changing the way you think… they're all amazingly effective strategies that will work – if you let them.

So, go – eat loads. And stay slim.

Best wishes, Peter

Della's Final Remarks

Today, my relationship with food is healthier than it's ever been. Today, I don't starve myself. I don't skip meals. I don't beat myself up or stress too much about my weight or get depressed about the odd flabby bit. I am also happy with what I see in my mirror – and I mean happy.

Part of that is, I suspect, because I am a little older and wiser than I used to be. I know I will never be twenty and effortlessly skinny again. But it's also because I know I don't have to do any of the heartbreakingly negative things I mentioned above.

Why not? Because I have the means to stay slim painlessly. I can, by making a few compromises in the way I eat, get on with living my life and enjoying my food and enjoying the fact that I have absolute control over the size of my jeans. Being in absolute control of what I eat is immensely freeing.

One of the bonuses of eating in the way that Peter and I have outlined in this book – and yes, I know we don't always agree, but we do agree on this one – is that we feel comfortable with ourselves.

I have discovered – and this still surprises me sometimes – that I actually prefer to eat what I have defined as smart choices for me. Maybe it's because I've retrained my taste buds. Or maybe it's because I know I can still have the odd bar of chocolate and I also know that no type of food is permanently denied to me.

Being slim, having the means to stay slim without stressing about it has changed my life in more ways than I ever thought possible. It can change yours too.

Happy planning.

All the very best, Della x

Disclaimer

Neither of the authors of this book have professional qualifications in nutrition. All advice contained within these pages is based upon the authors' personal experiences of losing weight, and/or their research of documentation freely available.

Please consult a medical professional before making radical changes to your diet.

If You've Enjoyed This Book…

(Peter and Della say…)

If you've enjoyed what you read and you'd like to 'spread the word', then here are a few ways you can do just that.

Review the book

Positive reviews are always welcome. Pop back to wherever you bought this book from to leave a glowing five star endorsement, or visit Amazon or Audible.

Like the Facebook Page

For starters, if you're on Facebook pop along to the Facebook page[18], and click the LIKE button (up there at the top).

Your 'friends' will be able to see that you're a fan, and you might see the occasional comments from other readers in your feed, as well as a daily post from us. Nothing too intrusive, we promise.

Feel free to post a comment or two yourself.

Follow us on Twitter

If you're more of a twitterer you can find us there under the handles @DellaGalton, @PeterJonesAuth, and @DoItAllBeHappy

---

[18] www.facebook.com/howtoeatloadsandstayslim

Got a blog or a podcast?

A mention of the book, or a link to the website (howtoeatloadsandstayslim.com) are always appreciated.

If you'd like either one of us to write a guest post for your blog, or interview either one of us for your podcast, just drop us a line.

Tell a friend

And finally, one of the hardest things for any author to achieve is 'word of mouth' recommendations. Next time you find yourself sitting next to someone who's telling you on and on how hard it is to enjoy food without piling on the pounds, do them, yourself, and us a favour – tell them about this book!

If you can do any of these things, we'd like to offer you our heartfelt thanks.

And whilst we're in the 'thanking' mood…

Acknowledgements

(Peter and Della say...)

In no particular order we'd really like to thank:

Jules – for everything you do, and not holding back whatsoever with your fantastic edits. Find out more about what Jules gets up to at balloonbaboon.co.uk

Author Wendy Steele – for her passion, advice and encouragement. Find out more about Wendy at WendySteele.com

Catherine King for her comments, feedback, encouragement and her lovely foreword.

Our completely brilliant agent, Becky Bagnell – for her unstoppable energy and enthusiasm, and for believing in us and this book. You can find her at lindsayliteraryagency.co.uk.

Alison the Proof Fairy – for once again stamping out any grammatical errors that dare to lurk between these pages (you can find her at theprooffairy.com).

Ellen for her fabulous cover design and artwork. Find out more about her at stalkandseed.com

To Kath at womagwriter.blogspot.co.uk for her endless support.

And to you, the reader. For taking a chance on this book and reading all the way to this point! You fabulously slender lovely person you.

Thank you all.

About Your Authors

Della Galton has been in the writing business for more than 25 years. She is a novelist, short story writer and journalist. She's had over a fifteen hundred short stories published in the UK alone and she's run out of fingers to count her books on.

She is a popular speaker at writing conventions and the agony aunt for Writers' Forum Magazine.

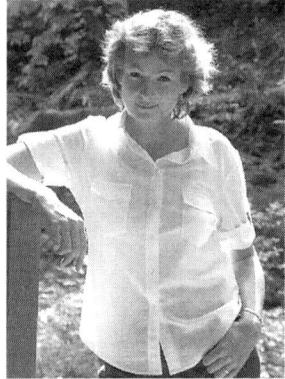

When Della isn't writing she enjoys walking her dogs around the beautiful Dorset countryside and beaches.

Find out more about Della,
her numerous books,
and her speaking engagements
at DellaGalton.co.uk

Peter Jones started professional life as a particularly rubbish graphic designer, followed by a stint as a mediocre petrol pump attendant. After that he got embroiled in the murky world of credit card banking. Fun times.

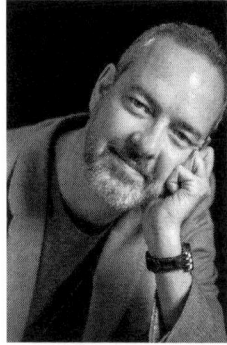

Now, Peter spends his days – most of them, anyway – writing.

He is the author of three and a half popular self-help books on the subjects of happiness, staying slim and dating. If you're overweight, lonely, or unhappy – he's definitely your guy.

His latest book "*The Good Guy's Guide to Getting The Girl*" is his début novel. It wasn't a 'historical' romance when he started out – it just took that long to write. The sequel is currently sitting on his desk. Waiting to be edited. Occasionally it seems to wink.

Peter doesn't own a large departmental store and probably isn't the same guy you've seen on the TV show Dragons' Den.

Find out more about Peter Jones,
his books, speaking engagements and workshops
at www.peterjonesauthor.com

Also In The Series

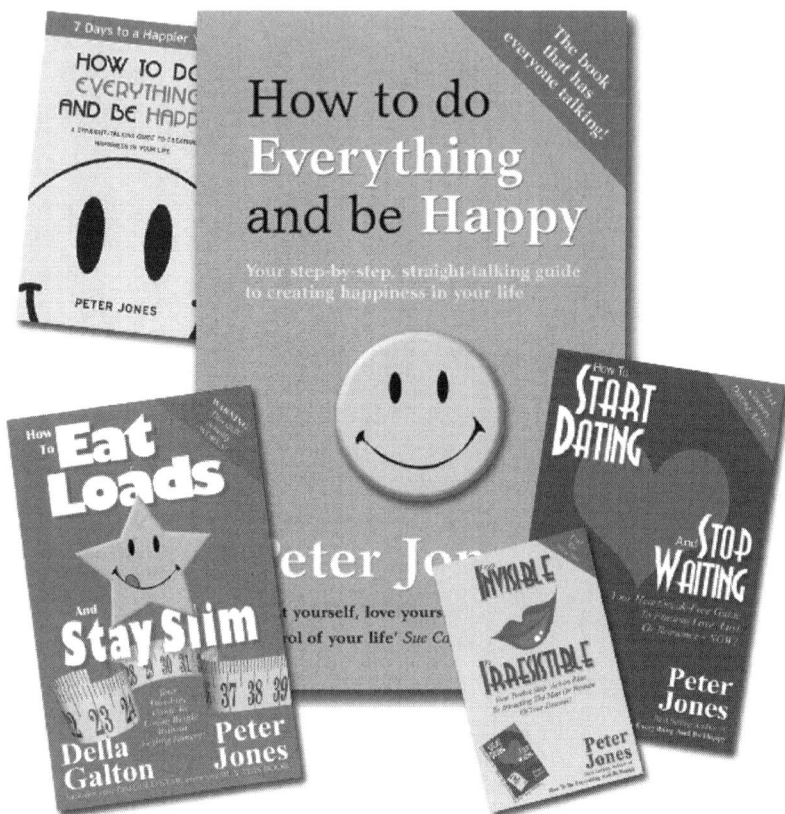

Change your life today…

It started with *How To Do Everything And Be Happy*, now it's a best-selling series. If you're unhappy, lonely or overweight, Peter Jones might just be the man for you

The books:

How To Do Everything And Be Happy
Your step-by-step, straight-talking guide to creating happiness in your life!

How To Eat Loads And Stay Slim
Your diet-free guide to losing weight without feeling hungry!

How To Start Dating And Stop Waiting
Your heartbreak-free guide to finding love, lust, or romance – now!

From Invisible To Irresistible
Your twelve step action plan to attracting the man or woman of your dreams!

Available in paperback,
for your e-reading device, or in audio.
Find out more at
www.HowToDoEverythingAndBeHappy.com

Also Available

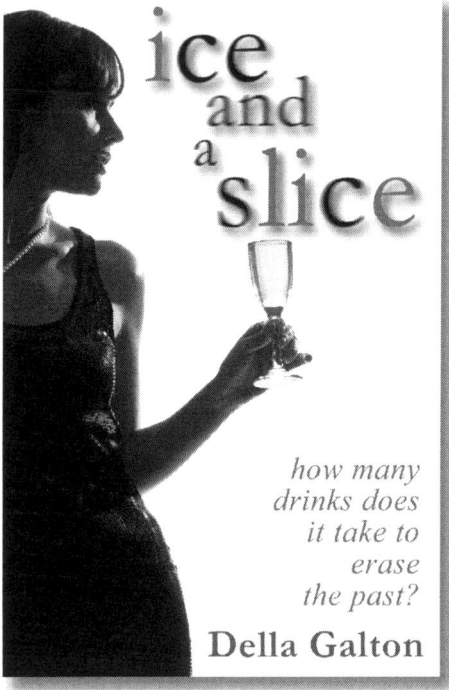

Ice And A Slice
The third full-length novel from
Della Galton

Ice And A Slice

Life should be idyllic, and it pretty much is for Sarah-Jane. Marriage to Tom is wonderful, even if he is hardly ever home. And lots of people have catastrophic fall-outs with their sister, don't they? They're bound to make it up some day. Just not right now, OK! And as for her drinking, yes it's true, she occasionally has one glass of wine too many, but everyone does that. It's hardly a massive problem, is it? Her best friend, Tanya, has much worse problems. Sarah-Jane's determined to help her out with them – just as soon as she's convinced Kit, the very nice man at the addiction clinic, that she's perfectly fine.

She is perfectly fine, isn't she?

Praise for Della's novels
"Della's writing is stylish, moving, original and fun : a wonderfully satisfying journey to a destination you can eagerly anticipate without ever guessing."
Liz Smith, Fiction Editor, My Weekly

Visit amazon to
buy the book
and find out more Della's fiction at
DellaGalton.co.uk

Also Available

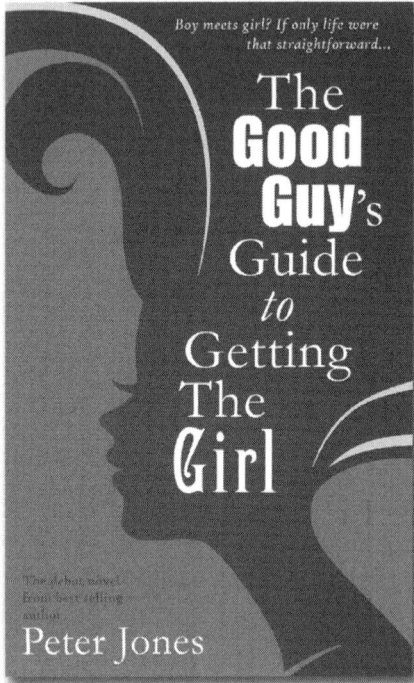

Boy meets girl? If only life were that straightforward...

The **Good Guy's** Guide *to* Getting The **Girl**

The debut novel from best selling author

Peter Jones

The Good Guy's Guide To Getting The Girl
The debut novel from
Peter Jones

The Good Guy's Guide
To Getting The Girl

"Liz. Where do I start?
I suppose the end is as good a place as any."

Boxing Day, 1997: Jason Smith, 29, and self-confessed 'good guy', is single again. And now that he is, it seems all the single girls – the 'Melanie Jacksons' of this world – are in short supply. Or are they? Has Jason stumbled on a foolproof way to find the girl of his dreams?

Both aided and hindered by his beer-drinking best buddy and reluctant father-to-be Alex, and his ever-wise, ever-sarcastic colleague Sian, 'The Good Guy's Guide to Getting The Girl' follows Jason on a voyage of self-discovery as he experiences the highs and lows of trying to meet one's soul mate at the turn of the millennium.

Visit amazon to
buy the book
and find out more Peter Jones at
PeterJonesAuthor.com

For a complete list of other great titles from
soundhaven books,
both fiction and non-fiction,
visit
www.soundhaven.com

9684042R00119

Printed in Great Britain
by Amazon.co.uk, Ltd.,
Marston Gate.